OTHER FAST FACTS BOOKS

Fast Facts About PTSD: A Guide for Nurses and Other Health Care Professionals (*Adams*)

Fast Facts for the NEW NURSE PRACTITIONER: What You Really Need to Know in a Nutshell, Second Edition (*Aktan*)

Fast Facts for the ER NURSE: Emergency Department Orientation in a Nutshell, Third Edition (*Buettner*)

Fast Facts About GI AND LIVER DISEASES FOR NURSES: What APRNs Need to Know in a Nutshell (*Chaney*)

Fast Facts for the MEDICAL–SURGICAL NURSE: Clinical Orientation in a Nutshell (*Ciocco*)

Fast Facts on COMBATING NURSE BULLYING, INCIVILITY, AND WORKPLACE VIOLENCE: What Nurses Need to Know in a Nutshell (*Ciocco*)

Fast Facts for the NURSE PRECEPTOR: Keys to Providing a Successful Preceptorship in a Nutshell (*Ciocco*)

Fast Facts for the OPERATING ROOM NURSE: An Orientation and Care Guide, Second Edition (*Criscitelli*)

Fast Facts for the ANTEPARTUM AND POSTPARTUM NURSE: A Nursing Orientation and Care Guide in a Nutshell (*Davidson*)

Fast Facts for the NEONATAL NURSE: A Nursing Orientation and Care Guide in a Nutshell (*Davidson*)

Fast Facts Workbook for CARDIAC DYSRHYTHMIAS AND 12-LEAD EKGs (*Desmarais*)

Fast Facts About PRESSURE ULCER CARE FOR NURSES: How to Prevent, Detect, and Resolve Them in a Nutshell (*Dziedzic*)

Fast Facts for the GERONTOLOGY NURSE: A Nursing Care Guide in a Nutshell (*Eliopoulos*)

Fast Facts for the LONG-TERM CARE NURSE: What Nursing Home and Assisted Living Nurses Need to Know in a Nutshell (*Eliopoulos*)

Fast Facts for the CLINICAL NURSE MANAGER: Managing a Changing Workplace in a Nutshell, Second Edition (*Fry*)

Fast Facts for EVIDENCE-BASED PRACTICE IN NURSING: Implementing EBP in a Nutshell, Third Edition (*Godshall*)

Fast Facts for Nurses About HOME INFUSION THERAPY: The Expert's Best Practice Guide in a Nutshell (*Gorski*)

Fast Facts About NURSING AND THE LAW: Law for Nurses in a Nutshell (*Grant, Ballard*)

Fast Facts for the L&D NURSE: Labor & Delivery Orientation in a Nutshell, Second Edition (*Groll*)

Fast Facts for the RADIOLOGY NURSE: An Orientation and Nursing Care Guide in a Nutshell (*Grossman*)

Fast Facts on ADOLESCENT HEALTH FOR NURSING AND HEALTH PROFESSIONALS: A Care Guide in a Nutshell (*Herrman*)

Fast Facts for the FAITH COMMUNITY NURSE: Implementing FCN/Parish Nursing in a Nutshell (*Hickman*)

Fast Facts for the CARDIAC SURGERY NURSE: Caring for Cardiac Surgery Patients in a Nutshell, Second Edition (*Hodge*)

Fast Facts About the NURSING PROFESSION: Histor

Fast Facts for the CLINICAL NURSING INSTRUCTOR Third Edition (*Kan, Stabler-Haas*)

Fast Facts for the WOUND CARE NURSE: Practical W

D1287439

Fast Facts About EKGs FOR NURSES: The Rules of Identifying EKGs in a Nutshell (*Landrum*)

Fast Facts for the CRITICAL CARE NURSE: Critical Care Nursing in a Nutshell (*Landrum*)

Fast Facts for the TRAVEL NURSE: Travel Nursing in a Nutshell (*Landrum*)

Fast Facts for the SCHOOL NURSE: School Nursing in a Nutshell, Second Edition (*Loschiavo*)

Fast Facts for MANAGING PATIENTS WITH A PSYCHIATRIC DISORDER: What RNs, NPs, and New Psych Nurses Need to Know (*Marshall*)

Fast Facts About SUBSTANCE USE DISORDERS: What Every Nurse, APRN, and PA Needs to Know (*Marshall, Spencer*)

Fast Facts About CURRICULUM DEVELOPMENT IN NURSING: How to Develop and Evaluate Educational Programs in a Nutshell, Second Edition (*McCoy, Anema*)

Fast Facts for the CATH LAB NURSE (*McCulloch*)

Fast Facts About NEUROCRITICAL CARE: A Quick Reference for the Advanced Practice Provider (*McLaughlin*)

Fast Facts for DEMENTIA CARE: What Nurses Need to Know in a Nutshell (*Miller*)

Fast Facts for HEALTH PROMOTION IN NURSING: Promoting Wellness in a Nutshell (*Miller*)

Fast Facts for STROKE CARE NURSING: An Expert Care Guide, Second Edition (*Morrison*)

Fast Facts for the MEDICAL OFFICE NURSE: What You Really Need to Know in a Nutshell (*Richmeier*)

Fast Facts for the PEDIATRIC NURSE: An Orientation Guide in a Nutshell (*Rupert, Young*)

Fast Facts About FORENSIC NURSING: What You Need to Know (*Scannell*)

Fast Facts About the GYNECOLOGICAL EXAM: A Professional Guide for NPs, PAs, and Midwives, Second Edition (*Secor, Fantasia*)

Fast Facts for the STUDENT NURSE: Nursing Student Success in a Nutshell (*Stabler-Haas*)

Fast Facts About RELIGION FOR NURSES: Implications for Patient Care (*Taylor*)

Fast Facts for CAREER SUCCESS IN NURSING: Making the Most of Mentoring in a Nutshell (*Vance*)

Fast Facts for the TRIAGE NURSE: An Orientation and Care Guide, Second Edition (*Visser, Montejano*)

Fast Facts for DEVELOPING A NURSING ACADEMIC PORTFOLIO: What You Really Need to Know in a Nutshell (*Wittmann-Price*)

Fast Facts for the HOSPICE NURSE: A Concise Guide to End-of-Life Care (*Wright*)

Fast Facts for the CLASSROOM NURSING INSTRUCTOR: Classroom Teaching in a Nutshell (*Yoder-Wise, Kowalski*)

Forthcoming FAST FACTS Books

Fast Facts About NEUROPATHIC PAIN: What Advanced Practice Nurses and Physician Assistants Need to Know (*Davies*)

Fact Facts in HEALTH INFORMATICS FOR NURSES (*Hardy*)

Fact Facts About NURSE ANESTHESIA (*Hickman*)

Fast Facts for the CARDIAC SURGERY NURSE, Third Edition (*Hodge*)

Fast Facts for the CRITICAL CARE NURSE: Critical Care Nursing, Second Edition (*Landrum*)

Fast Facts for the SCHOOL NURSE, Third Edition (*Loschiavo*)

Fast Facts on How to Conduct, Understand, and Maybe Even Love RESEARCH! For Nurses and Other Healthcare Providers (*Marshall*)

Fast Facts for DNP ROLE DEVELOPMENT: A Career Navigation Guide (*Menonna-Quinn, Genova*)

Fast Facts for MAKING THE MOST OF YOUR CAREER IN NURSING (*Redulla*)

Fast facts for the CLINICAL NURSE LEADER (*Wilcox, Deerhake*)

Visit www.springerpub.com to order.

FAST FACTS for
EVIDENCE-BASED
PRACTICE IN NURSING

Maryann Godshall, PhD, CCRN, CPN, CNE, is an associate clinical professor at Drexel University and a CCRN in the pediatric intensive care unit (PICU) at Lehigh Valley Health Network. At Drexel University, Dr. Godshall teaches adult critical care, pediatrics, pharmacology, and research. She has previously taught health and physical assessment, nursing concepts, evidence-based practice, and senior seminar. In addition, her responsibilities include syllabus development, management of course structure, administration of all grades, and facilitation of simulation experience. She previously taught at DeSales University, Cedar Crest College, Northampton Community College, and Lehigh County Community College. In addition to her clinical PICU experience at Lehigh Valley Health Network, Dr. Godshall currently works at Good Shepherd Inpatient Rehabilitation Hospital. Dr. Godshall has worked in PICU, pediatrics, pediatric home care, neonatal intensive care unit (NICU), and medical–surgical telemetry in a variety of hospital settings. She is one of the coeditors, with Dr. Ruth Wittmann-Price and Linda Wilson, of the *Certified Nurse Educator (CNE) Review Manual* (2017, Springer Publishing), for which she also authored a chapter. She has also written two chapters, "Caring for the Child With Cancer" and "Caring for the Child With a Chronic Condition or the Dying Child," and coauthored the chapter "Caring for a Child With an Integumentary Condition" in *Maternal–Child Nursing Care: Optimizing Outcomes for Mothers, Children, and Families*, edited by Susan L. Ward and Shelton M. Hisley. She has written a chapter on pediatric disaster preparedness, "Special Populations in Disasters: The Child and Pregnant Woman," in *Disaster Nursing: A Handbook for Practice*, edited by Deborah Adelman and Timothy J. Legg. She has published numerous journal articles and speaks both internationally and nationally on a variety of nursing topics. She has given three national poster presentations about both pediatric and nursing education topics. Her research topic was "Exploring Learning of Pediatric Burn Patients Through Storytelling," which she presented at the World Federation of Critical Care Nurses' 12th Congress in Brisbane, Australia, in 2016. She has also written NCLEX®-style questions in Kathryn Rudd and Diane Kocisko's *Davis Edge for Pediatric Nursing*, Second Edition, and the pediatric chapter in *NCLEX-RN® EXCEL: Test Success Through Unfolding Case Study Review*, Third Edition.

FAST FACTS for
EVIDENCE-BASED
PRACTICE IN NURSING

Third Edition

Maryann Godshall, PhD, CCRN, CPN, CNE

SPRINGER PUBLISHING COMPANY

Springer Publishing Company, LLC
11 West 42nd Street
New York, NY 10036
www.springerpub.com
http://connect.springerpub.com

Acquisitions Editor: Joseph Morita
Compositor: Amnet Systems

ISBN: 978-0-8261-6623-4
ebook ISBN: 978-0-8261-6624-1
DOI: 10.1891/9780826166241

19 20 21 22 / 5 4 3 2 1

The author and the publisher of this Work have made every effort to use sources believed to be reliable to provide information that is accurate and compatible with the standards generally accepted at the time of publication. Because medical science is continually advancing, our knowledge base continues to expand. Therefore, as new information becomes available, changes in procedures become necessary. We recommend that the reader always consult current research and specific institutional policies before performing any clinical procedure. The author and publisher shall not be liable for any special, consequential, or exemplary damages resulting, in whole or in part, from the readers' use of, or reliance on, the information contained in this book. The publisher has no responsibility for the persistence or accuracy of URLs for external or third-party Internet websites referred to in this publication and does not guarantee that any content on such websites is, or will remain, accurate or appropriate.

Library of Congress Cataloging-in-Publication Data

Names: Godshall, Maryann, author.
Title: Fast facts for evidence-based practice in nursing / Maryann Godshall.
Other titles: Fast facts for evidence-based practice.
Description: Third edition. | New York, NY: Springer Publishing Company,
   [2019] | Series: Fast facts | Includes bibliographical references and
   index.
Identifiers: LCCN 2019006138 (print) | LCCN 2019006829 (ebook) | ISBN
   9780826166241 (eBook) | ISBN 9780826166234 (alk. paper)
Subjects: | MESH: Evidence-Based Nursing—methods
Classification: LCC RT81.5 (ebook) | LCC RT81.5 (print) | NLM WY 100.7 | DDC
   610.73—dc23
LC record available at https://lccn.loc.gov/2019006138

Contact us to receive discount rates on bulk purchases.
We can also customize our books to meet your needs.
For more information please contact: sales@springerpub.com

Printed in the United States of America.

Contents

Preface

As a practicing nurse, I realize every day the importance of using the best evidence to deliver excellent-quality care to my patients. As an educator, I assist nurses in achieving their goal of obtaining their BSN. While teaching a course titled Evidence-Based Nursing Practice, I discovered that many of my students had never taken a basic research course. Indeed, they were fearful of research. I also had difficulty finding a suitable textbook that was written at the appropriate level and clearly explained the sometimes complex topics involved in research.

As a result, I decided to write my own book—one that nurses could use to understand basic research concepts, to assist them in obtaining "evidence" about their current daily practice, and to help them develop evidence-based practice (EBP) projects.

This book aims to assist both the experienced bedside nurse and the recent graduate in understanding EBP and in embracing its implementation as a means of improving the quality of patient care. For the bedside nurse, who may have significant clinical experience but may not have had the opportunity to take a research course, this book will serve as a guide to understanding the language and process of research. Alternatively, for the new nurse graduate, who may have taken a research course but may not have significant clinical experience, this book will serve as a useful reference in the workplace.

The book reviews the process of EBP, which involves defining a clinical situation of interest, formatting a good clinical question, conducting a literature search (i.e., finding the evidence), reading and critiquing research findings or published research reports (or both), and deciding if the evidence warrants a change in practice. This book also reviews basic research terms and principles.

The newly qualified nurse researcher may find this book useful in implementing new research to create evidence when none is yet available. It is my hope that this book will empower the reader to become comfortable with research reports and the research process and to embrace and use research to suggest enhancements to the quality of patient care in the clinical environment.

This book is organized to assist bedside nurses in understanding and developing EBP projects that relate to their patient populations. It delivers a wide scope of EBP content in the abbreviated style of the *Fast Facts* book series, developed by Springer Publishing. Short chapters offer key content using helpful headings and tables. "Fast Facts" boxes highlight important concepts and points in every chapter. Basic quantitative and qualitative research approaches are presented, as is an overview of EBP. This includes identifying the "compelling question," finding and critiquing the evidence, and exploring the importance of disseminating what you have found to your colleagues and professionals throughout the world. This book also attempts to demystify systemic reviews and to explain how to conduct database searches. The book has been classroom tested and used in both live and online course formats.

Maryann Godshall

ACKNOWLEDGMENTS

I would like to acknowledge all the bedside nurses who continue to strive for excellence by looking for the best evidence to provide the best clinical practice we can. I also would like to acknowledge the RN-to-BSN students in my EBP course, who were the reason this book was developed. The goal was to develop an EBP book to meet the needs of the typical bedside nurse that was quick and easy to use. I would like to thank Margaret Zuccarini, publisher emerita at Springer Publishing, who listened to my idea and encouraged me to write this book. I would also like to thank Hannah Hicks, assistant editor, and Joe Morita, senior acquisitions editor, at Springer Publishing, for their assistance in preparing this third edition and making it the best it can be. I would like to acknowledge Gary Childs for his helpful reviewing and assisting with up-to-date information in Chapter 7. Without all of these people, this dream would not have become a reality. Thank you all.

1

Introduction to Evidence-Based Practice

Every day, nurses are on the front line of patient care. It is the nurse who first notices a change in patient status. It is the nurse who implements and then evaluates the effectiveness of interventions. Often, nurses wonder who determines how nursing is practiced or why procedures are performed a certain way. A nurse might think, "It would be so much better if we did this procedure a different way." Did you ever wonder how you might change or influence the way patient care is delivered? New evidence comes into play every single day at the bedside as technology changes, research evolves, and patients present with new and unique disease processes. When nurses rely simply on the knowledge learned during their basic education their practice quickly becomes outdated. We have all evolved from simple patient care practitioners to nurse scientists. To be a proficient and informed nurse scientist, you need to remain current with the latest research and treatment modalities. Simply doing things "because we have always done them that way" is an outdated approach. Today, we must base our nursing and patient care on the latest evidence-based nursing research. If you have ever asked yourself such questions or wondered about practice issues, evidence-based practice (EBP) can be your road map to suggesting changes in the way patient care is delivered. It is the nurse who provides direct care to the patient. Why should not the nurse identify patient care problems and procedural issues, thereby recommending for consideration changes in how patient care is delivered? Now is the time for you to learn how you might use EBP strategies in your patient care area, unit, or institution.

In this chapter, you will learn:

1. The history of EBP
2. The definition of EBP
3. How to use EBP
4. An example of EBP
5. The requirements for EBP
6. Models of EBP
7. Controversies surrounding EBP
8. A rating system for the hierarchy of evidence in EBP
9. The limitations of EBP
10. EBP and Magnet® hospital designation

BRIEF HISTORY OF EBP

A cornerstone of the evidence-based movement was laid by Dr. Archie Cochrane, a British epidemiologist. Cochrane struggled with the efficacy of healthcare and challenged patients to pay only for care that was judged effective through proven methods. In 1972, Cochrane published a landmark book, *Effectiveness and Efficiency: Random Reflections on Health Services*, that criticized the medical profession for not conducting rigorous reviews of research evidence so that organizations and policy makers could reach valid decisions about healthcare. Cochrane strongly advocated determining preferred treatment and practice by using evidence from randomized clinical trials (RCTs). His support of the development of a system to systematically organize this information led to the creation of the Cochrane library (www.cochrane library.com). In 1993, **the Cochrane Collaboration was established to support international efforts to improve healthcare throughout the world**. More than 11,000 people have contributed to the collaboration (www.cochrane.org). Cochrane reviews bring together research on the effects of healthcare and are considered the gold standard for determining the effectiveness of different interventions.

Research Utilization and Nursing

During the 1980s, the field of nursing supported efforts to apply research findings to practice. This process, called **research utilization,** uses some aspect of a study in a manner unrelated to the intent of the original research. It may result in changing practice based only on the findings of a single research study (Barnsteiner & Prevost, 2002). Research utilization also focused on translating the existing research into practice instead of systematically determining the worthiness of findings of the research prior to implementing it into practice (Beyea & Slattery, 2013). **As research is conducted over time, evidence accumulates about a particular topic** (Polit & Beck, 2016) **that can be used to varying degrees in clinical practice.** For example, after reading a qualitative research article about the implications of hope for inpatients with long-term chronic illnesses, a nurse may be more aware of the importance of maintaining hope when working with these patients. As a result, the nurse may become more aware of how his or her actions may affect patients' feelings of hopefulness. **Through research utilization, the nurse may then change his or her actions** based on the reading of this one research article. **This may not have been the original intent of the research project.** Note that this example illustrates an instance in which the nurse demonstrates a greater awareness of the care he or she delivers. A nurse would not change the actual physical care of a patient without a change in an approved protocol, but a physician might.

The difference between research utilization and EBP is that **research utilization may lead to changes in practice that are based on the results of one study, whereas EBP answers a clinical question based on an in-depth literature search** conducted to find all relevant current research evidence related to that problem. So, although research utilization was an important concept to nursing, **the EBP movement has led to important changes in clinical actions and practice as a result of collaboration among the disciplines.** Today, most baccalaureate nursing programs have a required research course, which was not the case years ago.

Healthcare insurers and regulators have placed an emphasis on providing evidence-based care, especially where a cost savings can be found. The goal of improving care, decreasing costs, and promoting high-quality care should lead to shorter hospital stays and save insurance dollars. Healthcare institutions have focused on encouraging healthcare workers to develop methods for implementing evidence-based interventions, such as utilizing proper handwashing procedures to reduce the risk of transmission of microbes to patients (Beyea & Slattery, 2013).

Evolution From Research Utilization to EBP

Because EBP is broader than research utilization, nursing professionals began to actively explore the advantages of reviewing and analyzing all of the available evidence on a given topic or problem before taking steps to recommend a change in practice. Thus, **EBP represented a major paradigm shift for healthcare education and nursing practice**. As the profession of nursing has evolved, nurses have become more educated and involved in critiquing research studies. The purpose of critiquing is to analyze a study for flaws, evidence of bias, or other variables that might have affected the results. Polit and Beck (2016) note that a skillful clinician can no longer rely only on experience or a repository of memorized information, but he or she must now be adept in accessing, evaluating, synthesizing, and applying new research evidence.

Fast Facts

When evaluating research studies, make sure the research study design is congruent with its purpose. Quite simply, does the research study examine what it says it is going to?

Translating Research Into Practice

Translating research evidence into actual nursing practice is a challenging process. Some **resources are available to help implement EBP, including integrative reviews, systematic reviews, meta-analyses, and clinical practice guidelines (CPGs)**.

- **Integrative reviews** are scholarly papers that offer generalizations about substantive issues based on a set of relevant studies. They synthesize published studies and articles to find answers to questions of interest. They are frequently found in peer-reviewed professional publications (Mileham, 2009).
- A **systematic review** is a state-of-the-art summary of all the research information available at a given time on a particular subject. This is not a literature review but a review of actual research studies. All items in a systematic review address a specific clinical question. A systematic review attempts to cover all the evidence available. Systematic reviews can be found online at the websites of Joanna Briggs Institute (www.joannabriggs.org) and the Cochrane Collaboration Center (community.cochrane.org/handbook). The Cochrane Collaboration primarily addresses questions on the effectiveness of interventions or therapies and has a focus on synthesizing evidence from RCTs (Higgins & Green, 2011). The Briggs Institute includes other study designs and evidence derived from different sources in its systematic reviews (Aromataris

& Pearson, 2014). It is important to consider the source of a systematic review, particularly the credentials of the individual conducting the review and the integrity of the sources searched.

- A **meta-analysis** is a combination of the results of studies into a measurable format that statistically estimates the effects of proposed interventions and then critically reviews them to minimize bias. It is different from an integrative review in that it includes works that are similar or identical so that a statistical comparison can be made (Schmidt & Brown, 2009).

- **CPGs** are available to help guide clinical practice. As with systematic reviews, they distill a large amount of evidence into a manageable and usable format. **CPGs are practice recommendations based on the latest and best medical evidence available.** They can be used to guide clinical practice and clinical decision making that affects the diagnosis, treatment, prevention, or management of a particular medical issue or condition. This involves balancing the benefits and risks of an EBP decision. CPGs usually are based on systematic reviews and give specific practice recommendations and prescriptions for evidence-based decision making (Polit & Beck, 2016). CPGs are developed to help guide clinical practice even when only limited evidence is available. As multiple guidelines are being developed for the same topic, the same rigor must be used to critically appraise them as would be used in appraising a research article.

Fast Facts

Sources for CPGs include the Agency for Healthcare Research and Quality (https://www.ahrq.gov/gam/index.html), the Registered Nurses Association of Ontario (www.rnao.org/bestpractices), the Canadian Medical Association (www.cma.ca/En/Pages/clinical-practice-guidelines.aspx), and Translating Research into Practice (www.tripdatabase.com/index.html). There are also guides specific to such specialties as, for example, women's health and neonatal nursing.

EBP is based on a comprehensive review of research findings that emphasizes intervention, RCTs (the gold standard), integration of statistical findings, and critical decision making about the findings based on the strength of the evidence, tools used in the studies, and cost (Jennings, 2000; Jennings & Loan, 2001). Basic steps involved in implementing EBP are listed in Box 1.1.

Question: Do you have to be a nurse researcher to understand and utilize EBP?

Answer: No. EBP can be used by the bedside nurse to understand best clinical practices and to devise EBP projects of his or her own that may lead to recommendations for changes in clinical practices.

BOX 1.1   SEVEN STEPS OF EVIDENCE-BASED PRACTICE

1. Ask or identify the important clinical question.
2. Collect the best and most pertinent evidence.
3. Critically analyze and rate the evidence.
4. Integrate the evidence with your own clinical expertise, patient knowledge, and patient values in making a practice decision or recommending a change.
5. Implement your practice change, if authorized.
6. Evaluate how the practice change has influenced or affected your practice area.
7. Disseminate and share this evidence with your peers and colleagues.

Models of EBP

Several comprehensive models for implementing EBP have been developed. They include:

- ACE Star Model of Knowledge Transformation (Stevens, 2012)
- Advancing Research and Clinical Practice Through Close Collaboration (ARCC) Model (Melnyk & Fineout-Overholt, 2011)
- Clinical Nurse Scholar Model (Schultz, 2005)
- Diffusion of Innovations Theory (Rogers, 2003)
- Iowa Model of Evidence-Based Practice to Promote Quality Care (Titler et al., 2001)
- Johns Hopkins Nursing Evidence-Based Practice Model (Newhouse, Dearholt, Poe, Pugh, & White, 2007)
- Model for Change to Evidence-Based Practice (Rosswurm & Larrabee, 1999)
- Promoting Action on Research Implementation in Health Services (PARIHS) Model (Kitson et al., 2008)
- Stetler Model of Research Utilization (Stetler, 2001)

Steps and procedures in many of these models are similar; what differs is how these perspectives translate research into practice (Polit & Beck, 2016). Methods for implementing EBP and for asking the important clinical question are summarized in the following text and explored in detail in later chapters of this book.

DEFINITION OF EBP

The definition of EBP varies in relation to the concepts included. A search of the literature reveals that most definitions include (a) a focus on either the patient or the practitioner or (b) three components: research-based information, clinical expertise or practice, and patient care. Melnyk and Fineout-Overholt (2010) define EBP as an "approach that enables clinicians to provide the highest quality of care in meeting the multifaceted needs of patients and families" (p. 3). An article by Melnyk (2003) states that EBP is "a problem solving approach to clinical decision making that incorporates a search for the best and latest evidence, clinical expertise and assessment, and patient preference and values within a context of caring" (p. 149).

Sigma Theta Tau International (2005), in a position paper, defines evidence-based nursing as "an integration of the best evidence available, nursing expertise, and the values and preferences of the individuals, families and communities who are served." This takes into account not only the research-based evidence but also the situations nurses face when implementing best practices with people of various cultures, needs, and healthcare preferences. Sigma Theta Tau considers evidence-based nursing as a foundation for nursing practice.

Rutledge and Grant (2002) define EBP as "care that integrates best scientific evidence with clinical expertise, knowledge of pathophysiology, knowledge of psychosocial issues, and decision making preferences of patients" (p. 1). This definition expands EBP to include consideration of pathophysiology and psychosocial issues in the decision-making process. Magee (2005) directs the definition toward physician care versus nursing care and states that EBP is "the conscientious, explicit, and judicious use of current best evidence in making decisions about the care of the individual patients" (p. 73). Pravikoff, Tanner, and Pierce (2005) offer a simplified definition of EBP as "a systematic approach to problem solving for healthcare providers, including RNs, characterized by the use of the best evidence currently available for clinical decision-making in order to provide the most consistent and best possible care to patients" (p. 40). Ingersoll (2000) includes both the patient and the practitioner in her definition, stating that EBP is "the conscientious, explicit, and judicious use of theory driven research-based information in making decisions about care delivery to individuals or groups of patients and considers individual needs and preferences" (p. 152).

After considering these definitions, how can we define EBP for nursing? Quite simply, **EBP is using the best available evidence to guide clinical practice so that patients receive the best possible nursing care**. It is important to differentiate among the terms *evidence-based practice*, *evidence-based medicine*, and *evidence-based nursing*, as they should not be used interchangeably. Evidence-based medicine is how physicians practice medicine. EBP refers to physicians' or nurses' use of evidence to guide practice. Finally, evidence-based nursing emphasizes nursing interventions that are based on the best evidence.

HOW DO I PARTICIPATE IN AN EBP PROJECT?

Think of a clinical situation that generated questions in your mind for which you had no answers. There are several ways that you might try to find an answer to your question(s), including:

- Asking an authority or expert in the field
- Consulting a textbook
- Looking for an article in a nursing journal
- Looking for an article in a scholarly journal
- Asking a nursing peer or unit educator
- Using simple trial and error
- Using your intuition, judgment, or reasoning skills to solve the problem yourself

As you can see, these responses are varied. In nursing, especially if time is critical, nurses may be required to make the best judgment at a particular moment, but is this best practice? In making such a decision, does the nurse act in a routine manner in following accepted practice, or as an individual who takes the steps to find answers to questions, thereby promoting the knowledge base of nursing? **By using research evidence to guide practice, nurses can provide patients with the best interventions possible based on current research.**

EBP uses current research findings as the basis for practice rather than using "acceptable standards" of practice. In essence, the latter meant doing things because "that is how we have always done them." Nurses may make specific decisions in caring for patients because they have been taught that the expert nurses' experience "works the best." Those expert experiences are important and valued, but in the context of EBP they now are considered evidence that needs to be substantiated or validated through research and research dissemination in professional, scholarly, academic, and peer-reviewed publications. As the amount of evidence increases, so will EBP increase across professional nursing.

AN EXAMPLE OF EBP IN ACTION: SALINE VERSUS HEPARIN FLUSHES

Numerous studies have examined whether intermittent intravenous infusion reservoirs (heparin locks or wells) remain as patent with flushes of normal saline solution as with use of a heparin lock solution. Research evidence has demonstrated that saline flushes are as effective as heparin flushes for maintaining peripheral intermittent infusion devices using catheters larger than 24 gauge. This topic has been studied frequently in children. Lombardi, Gunderson, Zammett, Walters, and Morris (1988) conducted a sequential, nonrandom design of 74 catheter sites and found no difference in patency of catheters sized 20 to 24 gauge. In fact, there was a tendency for phlebitis to develop more often (13 vs. 7 sites in the normal saline group) with the use of heparin flush solutions. Danek and Noris (1992) examined 160 infusion devices and found no difference in patency of 22-gauge catheters. These findings were also supported by McMullen, Fioravanti, Pollack, Rideout, and Sciera (1993); Hanrahan, Kleiber, and Fagen (1994); and Robertson (1994). Beecroft, Bossert, and Chung (1997) carried out a collaborative study involving nine hospitals and 451 subjects and found that heparin-maintained (10 units/mL and 100 units/mL) catheters sized 22 and 24 gauge remained patent longer than did catheters that used saline alone as a flush. A randomized controlled trial by Mok, Kwon, and Chan (2007), two of whom are clinical nurses and one a nursing professor, found no significant differences in the longevity of catheter patency or incidence of intravenous complications of 123 intravenous locks maintained with saline flush or heparin flush (1 unit/mL or 10 units/mL).

Now, if you ask who first questioned the practice of using heparin flushes or whether saline flushes might be as effective as heparin flushes, you will learn that it was a nurse. This is just one example of how a nurse's observations and subsequent questioning changed nursing practice. Your observations or ideas, too, can change practice by initiating the question, conducting a literature review based on that question, examining the evidence, and, if no evidence exists, suggesting that research studies might be needed to create the evidence to substantiate your hunch or idea.

As a nurse embarking on EBP, it is important for you to first understand the basic concepts of research and how to rate or evaluate the evidence before suggesting that it be used to guide practice. Understanding nursing research will enable you to better apply research findings in your everyday practice.

REQUIREMENTS FOR AN EBP STUDY

The move toward EBP means, by definition, that anyone can conduct an exhaustive search of the literature and analyze the findings to determine the best evidence. **A hospital librarian or nursing colleague can assist you in getting started to find research articles.** A novice, who does not have the background or perhaps does not understand basic research methods, should ask a more experienced mentor for assistance in evaluating such research. Always remember that an EBP project requires an exhaustive, systematic, and analytical review of the literature. Although a single study should never result in a change in practice, the results of one study might provide the impetus to look at a current clinical process, construct a clinical question, and conduct further research that might support or invalidate the findings of that one study.

The seasoned nurse must use sound reasoning and clinical judgment. Benner, Tanner, and Chesla (2009) describe clinical judgment as the way in which nurses come to understand and respond in concerned and involved ways based on salient information in a situation. Clinical judgment should encourage use of all types of available knowledge on which decisions can be based. The nurse's knowledge of patients or clients as people takes into consideration both cultural and ethical values in every step of the nursing process (Benner et al., 2009). For example, although research might show that a particular intervention is effective in reducing complications of stroke, this same intervention might not be acceptable in populations whose religious or cultural beliefs oppose this type of intervention.

CONTROVERSIES SURROUNDING EBP

EBP as a "Cookbook" Approach to Care

One controversy about EBP is that it offers a so-called cookbook approach to care and may override the individualization of care.

Fast Facts

One research study should never change nursing clinical practice. A researcher must perform a complete review of the literature and then analyze the findings to determine if this evidence has merit and should actually change practice.

Clinical decisions should be based on the evidence as well as on a response to specific clinical situations or patients (Melnyk & Fineout-Overholt, 2015). It could also be argued that EBP might discourage attention to cultural issues, but nursing care must consider cultural variations in every given situation.

No Evidence

Another important controversy surrounding EBP is that no evidence may exist pertaining to a particular clinical question or that the purported evidence or research published on the clinical topic of interest may be weak, poorly structured, or flawed. Another concern is that existing evidence may be too limited to serve as the basis for changing practice. For some topics of interest, there may be just one published research study. While you may be excited to find research on your topic of interest, it is important to critically evaluate the research that you have found. How do you conduct a critical evaluation to determine if it is good research? There are protocols to follow when evaluating research. If the research is not considered "good"—that is, reliable—then there is a need for a research study to be conducted on your clinical question so that good evidence can be generated and published.

Randomized Clinical Trials

Some experts argue that because an RCT is the gold standard for evaluating EBP results, other research methods should essentially be ignored. Using this reasoning, qualitative research studies that yield valid and important evidence in exploring the problem under consideration might be disregarded in place of an RCT. However, integration of evidence relevant to nursing practice is a key component of EBP. Nurses must pay attention to all types and levels of evidence and not simply look for or use only RCTs, even though they are considered the highest level of evidence. In addition, the prudent nurse researcher should consider evidence from all disciplines as well as all types of research methodology, to gain a thorough understanding of

BOX 1.2 RATING SYSTEM FOR HIERARCHY OF EVIDENCE

Level 1: Evidence from a systematic review or meta-analysis of all relevant RCTs or established EBP clinical guidelines

Level 2: Evidence obtained from at least one well-designed RCT

Level 3: Evidence obtained from a well-designed controlled trial without randomization or a systematic review of correlational/observational studies

Level 4: Evidence from well-designed case-control and cohort studies that are correlational or observational

Level 5: Evidence from systematic reviews of descriptive, qualitative, or physiological studies

Level 6: Evidence from a single descriptive, qualitative, or physiological study

Level 7: Evidence from the opinion of authorities/experts or case reports of expert committees, or both

EBP, evidence-based practice; RCT, randomized clinical trial.

Source: Adapted from Melnyk B. M., & Fineout-Overholt, E. (2010). *Evidence-based practice in nursing & healthcare: A guide to best practice* (2nd ed.). Philadelphia, PA: Lippincott Williams & Wilkins; Polit, D. G., & Beck, C. T. (2016). *Nursing research: Generating and assessing evidence for nursing practice* (10th ed.). Philadelphia, PA: Wolters Kluwer.

the available literature on the clinical question. The hierarchy and rating system for evaluating research evidence is provided in Box 1.2.

Finally it might be argued that EBP does not consider nursing theory as well as humanistic aspects of care. For those interested in nursing theory, very few research studies are based on or use nursing theory. This is another issue and concern voiced by the nursing profession.

EBP and Magnet Hospital Designation

Twenty-five years ago, the American Nurses Credentialing Center (ANCC) developed the Magnet Recognition Program as a way of highlighting healthcare organizations that achieve a hallmark of excellence for nursing practice and professional development. To attain Magnet status, hospitals must demonstrate quality nursing care through EBP. This includes patient care delivery that is guided by the integration of best evidence, clinical care decisions based on critical thinking, and improved patient outcomes. EBP committees have emerged as a way to provide a systematic approach for enabling new evidence to reach the bedside nurse. For ANCC Magnet reapplication, the focus is placed more strongly on clinical outcomes. The Magnet program encourages nurses to guide their clinical practice and make recommendations. An EBP committee becomes the best mechanism for integrating best evidence into clinical practice settings and keeps nurses actively involved in improving patient outcomes (Wise, 2009).

The growth of nurse residency programs in the United States to assist the transition of new graduate nurses into the profession has grown in popularity. Many of these nurse residency programs require the development of an EBP project. This will be discussed in Chapter 10, Evidence-Based Practice in the Nurse Residency Program.

LIMITATIONS OF EBP

Limitations of EBP include a shortage of good, coherent, and consistent scientific evidence in support of nursing practice. There is also difficulty in applying the evidence obtained to individual patients in particular clinical situations (Fain, 2009). Some nurses are hesitant or might even refuse to consider using EBP in their nursing practice and care. It is important to understand why this occurs. **The reasons nurses give for not using research findings in their clinical practices are listed in Box 1.3.**

Fast Facts

Pravikoff et al. (2005), in a report entitled "Readiness of U.S. Nurses for Evidence-Based Practice," summarized their findings from a random sample of 3,000 nurses in the United States. They concluded that while RNs generally acknowledge the need for information in order to assure effective practice, they simply were not prepared to use the information resources available to them.

BOX 1.3   REASONS WHY NURSES DO NOT USE RESEARCH FINDINGS IN THEIR PRACTICES

1. Nurses may not know about or be aware of research findings.
2. Nurses in practice do not usually associate or communicate with those who produce research findings.
3. Nurses lack the ability to locate and find relevant research reports.

(continued)

BOX 1.3   REASONS WHY NURSES DO NOT USE RESEARCH FINDINGS IN THEIR PRACTICES (*continued*)

4. Research is often in language that is not clinically meaningful.
5. Nurses do not understand research methods and have never had formal research classes in their nursing schools.
6. Nurses lack the value for research in practice.
7. Computer databases are not readily accessible to the nurse.
8. Nurses lack the basic knowledge to use information technology.
9. Nurses have no time to obtain this information.
10. Nurses do not understand exactly what EBP is.
11. People have a fear of the unknown and a fear of change. By understanding these processes, fear can be alleviated.

EBP, evidence-based practice.

Source: Adapted from Fain, J. A. (2009). *Reading, understanding, and applying nursing research* (3rd ed.). Philadelphia, PA: F. A. Davis; Pravikoff, D. S., Tanner, A. B., & Pierce, S. T. (2005). Readiness of U.S. nurses for evidence-based practice. *American Journal of Nursing, 105*(9), 40–51. doi:10.1097/00000446-200509000-00025

The reasons why RNs were generally unprepared for EBP include:

- Limited time availability
- Little or no education or training in information retrieval or accessing computer databases
- Lack of needed basic computer skills
- Limited access to high-quality information resources or databases
- Attitudes that did not value or understand research

Pravikoff and colleagues (2005) felt this could be attributed to the rapid technological changes over the past 10 to 15 years, along with the failure of nursing education programs to prepare students at all levels to understand and value research-based practice versus a practice based on tradition, intuition, and nursing experience.

Fast Facts

So, now is the time for you to learn about basic research principles and to increase your understanding of what EBP is all about. This book will guide you in unlocking the mysteries of EBP and help you understand how evidence can be used in your clinical area to change or improve practice. Let's get started in determining how EBP can be used by working through some examples of how an evidence-based project might begin.

Once you have explored the beginnings of an EBP project in the next few chapters, you will learn why it is important to pay careful attention to overcoming the barriers to implementing EBP. Methods and suggestions to do so will be discussed in detail in Chapter 8, Evaluating the Evidence.

REFERENCES

Aromataris, E., & Pearson, A. (2014). A systematic review: An overview. *American Journal of Nursing, 114*(3), 53–58. doi:10.1097/01.NAJ.0000444496.24228.2c

Barnsteiner, J., & Prevost, S. (2002). How to implement evidence-based practice: Some tried and true pointers. *Reflections on Nursing Leadership, 28*(2), 18–21.

Beecroft, P. C., Bossert, E., & Chung, K. (1997). Intravenous lock patency in children: Dilute heparin versus saline. *Journal of Pediatric Pharmacology Practice, 2*(4), 211–223.

Benner, P., Tanner, C. A., & Chesla, C. A. (Eds.). (2009). *Expertise in nursing practice: Caring, clinical judgment and ethics* (2nd ed.). New York, NY: Springer Publishing.

Beyea, S., & Slattery, M. J. (2013). Historical perspectives on evidence based nursing. *Nursing Science Quarterly, 26*(2), 152–155. doi:10.1177/0894318413477140

Danek, G. D., & Noris, E. M. (1992). Pediatric IV catheters: Efficacy of saline flush. *Pediatric Nursing, 18*(2), 111–113.

Fain, J. A. (2009). *Reading, understanding, and applying nursing research* (3rd ed.). Philadelphia, PA: F. A. Davis.

Hanrahan, K. S., Kleiber, C., & Fagan, C. (1994). Evaluation of saline for IV locks in children. *Pediatric Nursing, 20*(6), 549–552.

Higgins, J. P. T., & Green, S. (2011, March) *Cochrane handbook for systematic reviews of interventions* (Version 5.1.0). Retrieved from http://community.cochrane.org/handbook

Ingersoll, G. L. (2000). Evidence-based nursing: What it is and what it isn't. *Nursing Outlook, 48*(4), 151–152. doi:10.1067/mno.2000.107690

Jennings, B. W. (2000). Evidence-based practice: The road best traveled? *Research in Nursing and Health, 23*(5), 343–345. doi:10.1002/1098-240X(200010)23:53.0.CO;2-7

Jennings, B. W., & Loan, L. A. (2001). Misconceptions among nurses about evidence-based practice. *Journal of Nursing Scholarship, 33*(2), 121–127. doi:10.1111/j.1547-5069.2001.00121.x

Kitson, A., Rycroft-Malone, J., Harvey, G., McCormack, B., Seers, K., & Titchen, A. (2008). Evaluating the successful implementation of evidence into practice using the PARiHS framework: Theoretical and practical challenges. *Implementation Science, 3*(1), 1–12. doi:10.1186/1748-5908-3-1

Lombardi T. P., Gunderson, B., Zammett, L. O., Walters, J. K., & Morris, B. A. (1988). Efficacy of 0.9% sodium chloride injection with or without heparin sodium for maintaining patency of intravenous catheters in children. *Clinical Pharmacology, 7*(11), 832–836.

Magee, M. (2005). *Health politics: Power, population and health*. Bronxville, NY: Spencer Books.

McMullen, A., Fioravanti, I. D., Pollack, V., Rideout, K., & Sciera, M. (1993). Heparinized saline or normal saline as a flush solution in intermittent intravenous lines in infants and children. *American Journal of Maternal/Child Nursing, 18*(2), 78–85. doi:10.1097/00005721-199303000-00005

Melnyk, B. M. (2003). Finding and appraising systematic reviews of clinical interventions: Critical skills for evidence-based practice. *Pediatric Nursing, 29*(2), 147–149.

Melnyk, B. M., & Fineout-Overholt, E. (2010). *Evidence-based practice in nursing & healthcare: A guide to best practice* (2nd ed.). Philadelphia, PA: Lippincott Williams & Wilkins.

Melnyk, B. M., & Fineout-Overholt, E. (2011). The ARCC model and role of EBP mentors in promoting professional practice attributes. Presented at Sigma Theta Tau International Conference. Phoenix, AZ: Arizona State University.

Melnyk, B. M., & Fineout-Overholt, E. (2015). *Evidence-based practice in nursing & health care: A guide to best practice* (3rd ed.). Philadelphia, PA: Wolters Kluwer.

Mileham, P. (2009). Finding sources of evidence. In N. Schmidt & J. Brown (Eds.), *Evidence-based practice: Appraisal and application of research* (pp. 75–82). Boston, MA: Jones & Bartlett.

Mok, E., Kwon, T., & Chan, M. F. (2007). A randomized controlled trial for maintaining peripheral intravenous infusion devices in children. *International Journal of Nursing Practice, 13*(1), 33–45. doi:10.1111/j.1440-172X.2006.00607.x

Newhouse, R. P., Dearholt, S. L., Poe, S. S., Pugh, L. C., & White, K. M. (2007). *Johns Hopkins guidelines to evidence based practice: Models & guidelines*. Indianapolis, IN: Sigma Theta Tau International.

Polit, D. G., & Beck, C. T. (2016). *Nursing research: Generating and assessing evidence for nursing practice* (10th ed.). Philadelphia, PA: Wolters Kluwer.

Pravikoff, D. S., Tanner, A. B., & Pierce, S. T. (2005). Readiness of U.S. nurses for evidence-based practice. *American Journal of Nursing, 105*(9), 40–51. doi:10.1097/00000446-200509000-00025

Robertson, J. (1994). Intermittent intravenous therapy: A comparison of two flushing solutions. *Contemporary Nursing, 3*(4), 174–179. doi:10.5172/conu.3.4.174

Rogers, E. M. (2003). *Diffusions of innovations* (5th ed.). New York, NY: Simon & Schuster.

Rosswurm, M. A., & Larrabee, J. H. (1999). A model for change to evidence-based practice. *Image: The Journal of Nursing Scholarship, 31*(4), 317–322. doi:10.1111/j.1547-5069.1999.tb00510.x

Rutledge, D. N., & Grant, M. (2002). Introduction. *Seminars in Oncology Nursing, 18*, 1–2. doi:10.1053/sonu.2002.37404

Schmidt, N. A., & Brown, J. M. (2009). *Evidence-based practice for nurses: Appraisal and application of research.* Sudbury, MA: Jones & Bartlett.

Schultz, A. (2005). Clinical scholars at the bedside: An EBP mentorship model for today. *Journal of Excellence in Nursing Knowledge, 2*(2), 1–8.

Sigma Theta Tau International. (2005). *Evidence based nursing position statement.* Indianapolis, IN: Author. Retrieved from https://www.sigmanursing.org/why-sigma/about-sigma/position-statements-and-resource-papers/evidence-based-nursing-position-statement

Stetler, C. B. (2001) Updating the Stetler Model of research utilization to facilitate evidence-based practice. *Nursing Outlook, 49*(6), 272–279. doi:10.1067/mno.2001.120517

Stevens, K. R. (2012). ACE Star model of EBP: Knowledge transformation. Academic Center for Evidence-Based Practice. The University of Texas Health Science Center. Retrieved from http://nursing.uthscsa.edu/onrs/starmodel/star-model.asp

Titler, M. G., Kleiber, C., Steelman, V., Rakel, B., Budreau, G., & Everett, L. (2001). The Iowa model of evidence based practice to promote quality care. *Critical Care Nursing Clinics of North America, 13*(4), 497–509. doi:10.1016/S0899-5885(18)30017-0

Wise, N. J. (2009). Maintaining magnet status: Establishing an evidence based practice committee. *AORN Journal, 90*(2), 205–213. doi:10.1016/j.aorn.2009.02.016

2

Asking the Compelling Question

When beginning an evidence-based practice (EBP) project, several steps are crucial to consider, including developing a well-constructed clinical question. Taking time to construct a clinical question is of chief importance because this question will drive every aspect of your research, from the initial literature search to the final success of your project. This chapter explains how to begin selecting your clinical question and provides tools to construct a high-quality clinical question.

In this chapter, you will learn:

1. How to start an EBP project
2. How to structure a compelling clinical question
3. How to use the PICOT method in implementing EBP
4. How to determine if a study is valid and reliable

HOW TO START AN EBP PROJECT

Sackett, Straus, Richardson, Rosenberg, and Hayes (2000) described this step as the most challenging in the EBP process. Where do you find an appropriate question? **Your clinical or work environment presents many opportunities for developing a compelling question**, such as those listed here.

- Has there been a time in clinical practice when you wondered, "Why do we do it this way," and, after asking a colleague, received the answer, "Because that is the way we have always done it" or "Because that is the only way it works"? The next time you hear these words, take a step back and ask yourself, "Does this make sense?"

- Why do nurses always use a black pen to chart their notes? Is it simply preference or the result of trial and error? The reason is simple. When photocopying and scanning notes into the computer database, black ink shows up better than blue. This illustrates a trial-and-error method of problem solving, but it also provides a relevant example of a possible source of a compelling clinical question.

- Have you wondered why bed alarms are used for particular patients? The answer is that a research study showed that bed alarms decreased the number of patient falls on a given unit. A screening tool identified patients considered to be "at risk." For these patients, a bed alarm was activated, and the fall risk for those patients was reduced. This sounds quite basic, but several research studies have shown the effectiveness of bed alarms in decreasing patient falls. This nursing practice is a good example of EBP.

Other areas to consider when searching for a compelling clinical question include etiology, diagnoses, therapies, prevention strategies, and prognoses. Questions you might consider are those that provide meaning or insight into a phenomenon that might help nurses to appreciate or relate to a patient's experience or to understand the growing impact of culture on the administration of healthcare today. With the skyrocketing cost of healthcare, the question could also include a cost-containment measure or an intervention that could decrease the length of a patient's stay in the hospital. All of these are areas for an inquisitive mind to explore.

Current research studies usually conclude with a summary discussion and a section describing the implications for further research. These are both potential sources of ideas for clinical questions. Thus, if you have the experience and qualifications, your initial EBP project may enable you to design and conduct your own research study. It is perfectly acceptable to build on existing research and answer a question posed by another author. This can be a **research problem** that is an area of concern or that illustrates a gap in current knowledge or in the literature. This research problem can also be the impetus to helping to form your EBP clinical question.

In developing an EBP project, one could also consider questions that might build on current nursing theory. Investigate national initiatives by U.S. government agencies, some of which routinely identify health problems and sometimes suggest research priorities. Topical areas suggested by authors for further investigation do not necessarily have to develop into full research studies, but they can inspire an EBP project. This is particularly true if it proves to be an area that might save a healthcare agency money or improve a process. Some excellent places to start might be the research agendas for health concerns (Adams, 2009), examples of which are available on the following government websites:

- U.S. Surgeon General's Office (www.surgeongeneral.gov)
- National Institutes of Health (www.nih.gov)
- National Institute of Nursing Research (www.ninr.nih.gov)
- National Institute of Mental Health (www.nimh.nih.gov)

Who knows? Your EBP project could develop into a research study.

The clinical question you develop will most likely fall into one of the following categories:

- Diagnosis identification or recognition
- Therapy or intervention
- Etiology
- Impact of the prognosis
- Prevention strategy

HOW TO STRUCTURE THE COMPELLING QUESTION IN A SEARCHABLE AND ANSWERABLE FORMAT

When asking a compelling question, be sure the question is phrased so that it can be answered. If it is worded too broadly, you may not be able to find a usable answer. Simply restating the question may sometimes solve this problem. For example, perhaps you wanted to ask, "Why are patients angry?" Although this is a good question, it really is too broad to answer meaningfully or specifically. A better question would be, "Are anger levels lower in patients admitted to the ED as compared with patients admitted directly to the medical surgical floor?" Now you have narrowed your focus to a comparison between anger levels in patients being admitted to two different units. This is much more specific. The environment in which they are placed may or may not play a part in their anger. The more specific your question is, the more answerable it becomes.

Another consideration is the amount of evidence available to answer your question. If a lot of evidence exists, your question may already have been asked multiple times and does not need to be asked again. If this might be the situation in relation to your question, move on to another question. On the other hand, if no evidence is available to support your question, you may have identified an important question that should be explored. Where will you begin to find the evidence to support a question that has never been asked? First, you might look to the field of medicine for relevant studies and then to related disciplines.

For example, you might decide to investigate the stress a family member experiences when walking into the ICU for the first time. If you can find no nursing studies on this topic, you should look at resources in psychology that explore stress and coping theory. While these studies may not have been conducted in the intensive care environment, they relate by focusing on the human reaction to stress.

THE PICOT FORMAT

Many methods are available for implementing EBP projects. One simple method used in this book is the PICOT format, presented by Melnyk and Fineout-Overholt (2010).

Fast Facts

The PICOT acronym is broken down as follows:

P = Patient or Population of interest
I = Intervention of interest
C = Comparison of interest
O = Outcome of interest
       Initially only four components were included. Later, Melnyk and Fineout-Overholt added a fifth, representing time (i.e., the time it takes for the intervention to achieve an outcome, or how long participants are observed).
T = Time it takes to demonstrate an outcome

Step One: Defining the Patient Population of Interest

The first step in formulating a research or EBP question is to decide what **population** you want to examine. Are you interested in infants, children, adults, or geriatric individuals? Perhaps you are interested in people with psychological disorders or people with whom you deal in the community. In defining the population, describe the group clearly. If you are interested in studying the geriatric group, what ages will you include in your group: people older than 50, 55, 60, or

65 years? Will your group include male or female patients, or both? If you are interested in working with children, what group will you include: infants, toddlers, preschoolers, school-age children, or adolescents? Will your group include boys or girls, or both? Be very clear when defining your population of interest.

The reason the patient population must be carefully described is that you want the search engines to give you relevant information and not information that is too broad or off target. (This will be discussed further in Chapter 6, Qualitative Research.) When retrieving information in a literature search, keep in mind that research findings reported for one patient population may not be relevant to another (Adams, 2009). For example, if you are looking at the effects of thrombolytic agents in children and you find a study that examines thrombolytic agents in adults, you cannot assume that the thrombolytic agents will work the same in different patient populations. This is only one of many important variables to consider that can affect any study.

Fast Facts

When looking at a particular population of interest, be sure to consider age, gender, race, ethnicity, disease process, comorbid conditions, and any characteristic that may affect the chosen population.

Step Two: Identifying the Intervention or Process of Interest

The second step is to decide what **intervention** or **process** you want to examine. What do you want to do for this patient population? Ask yourself these questions:

- Have I ever asked why nurses follow a particular process, without receiving a logical answer?
- Have I found that performing an intervention in one particular way seems to be more effective than another?
- Have I seen patients improve and recover more quickly when a particular intervention has been used?
- Have I noticed that when a particular physician is on call, the patients do better—or worse—in relation to a particular intervention?
- Have I noticed that the unit seems to have a large number of infected central lines, or sepsis?
- Have I noticed that the unit seems to be calmer when certain individuals are working and less controlled when other

individuals are present? Why? Is there something different in the care delivered?

- Have I noticed that there might be a better and more cost-effective way to perform an intervention I do every day?
- Do I feel that practice standards in a particular area are lacking?
- Have I recently read an article about a particular topic and thought, "Hey, that is a good idea" or "Why do we not do that in my unit?"

These are just some questions that could be the impetus for finding a better way, or justifying an existing way, in which nursing practice and interventions are performed. Quite simply, ask yourself what burning question or pet peeve you have or what does not make sense when performing your daily nursing routine? What do you feel could be done better? Is there something you feel is wasteful and could be done a different way to decrease costs, improve patient outcomes, or reduce time required? Table 2.1 contains information to consider when looking at each of these questions.

In researching an intervention or treatment, remember to compare the reaction of individuals who receive the intervention with the reaction of individuals who do not receive the treatment. If the latter group received a placebo, the effect of that placebo must also be considered. Patients who receive a placebo, or harmless intervention, think they have received the actual treatment. As such, they constitute a control group against which the patients receiving the actual intervention can be measured. If, for example, the subjects who received a sugar pill experience any "effects," they are known as "placebo effects." The more defined the intervention is, the more focused your question will be, which will help avoid any placebo effects.

Step Three: Examining the Comparison of Interest

The comparison of interest is the alternative to your intervention. The comparison can be a **control (no treatment) versus a placebo (fake treatment)**. The comparison can also consist of **measuring your intervention of interest against what is considered to be the gold standard** of treatment for a particular situation or disease process.

Suppose, for example, that you plan to study a fall intervention strategy in an elderly population. First, you would want to learn what the literature says about fall interventions in your patient population. Then, you might conduct a minisurvey of your patient population

Table 2.1

The PICOT Method for Implementing Evidence-Based Practice Projects

Patient population of interest	The patient population for the problem of interest: ■ Age ■ Gender ■ Ethnicity ■ Educational status ■ With certain disease process or disorder (e.g., heart disease, diabetes, pancreatitis)
Intervention	The intervention or interventions of interest: ■ Exposure to disease ■ Prognostic factor A ■ Risk behaviors (e.g., smoking, drug usage, cholesterol levels)
Comparison	What you want to compare the intervention to or against: ■ No disease ■ Placebo or no intervention ■ Type of therapy given or not ■ Prognostic factor B ■ Absence of a risk factor or characteristic (e.g., a nonsmoker, non–drug user)
Outcome	Outcome of interest, what is the result? ■ Risk of disease ■ Accuracy of diagnosis ■ Rate of occurrence of adverse outcome (e.g., severe illness, development of a comorbid condition, or even death)
Time	Time it takes to demonstrate an outcome (the time it takes for the intervention to achieve an outcome, or how long participants are observed)

and fall interventions. Finally, you could compare your fall intervention strategy group to a group of elderly patients who do not receive that specific intervention. You could also do a simple performance improvement (PI) or quality assurance (QA) survey of your patient population. This does not have to involve a large group. You could then compare what you found in the literature with what you found on your unit. The resulting data can be impressive and are particularly useful when approaching the institution's administration to consider implementing a practice change. Although a survey is not necessary—you could just present the evidence—including survey data from your institution's patient population in addition to the review of the literature results in a stronger presentation.

Another example is the use of pain medication in the pediatric population. One group could receive a narcotic medication in the form of a lollipop (e.g., Fentanyl lollipops), while the other group does not. The comparison of interest would be an evaluation of any difference in the level of pain experienced by the two groups. Again, you would search the literature first and then conduct an informal survey of your patients. Keep in mind which patients are receiving such medications and which patients are undergoing which procedures. As this step may go beyond a simple survey of your patient population, it may require administrative and institutional review board (IRB) approval. Always check with your hospital administration before embarking on any type of data collection procedures to be sure you are operating within institutional policy guidelines and maintaining patient confidentiality.

To adjust the preceding example to compare the type of intervention, consider whether one group of children received the narcotic lollipop and another group received a regular lollipop without medication in it. The comparison of interest would be whether the groups experienced different levels of pain. In this example, you would need to use the same developmentally appropriate pain scale to measure pain in both groups. This would be a 0 to 10 scale for older adolescent children and, perhaps, the Wong-Baker FACES® Pain Rating Scale for school-age children.

Step Four: Outcome of Interest

The last step is establishing the outcome of interest. What will be improved, or what do you want to see happen to the patient? **What do you want to accomplish or measure?** The *Cochrane Handbook for Systematic Review of Interventions* (Higgins & Green, 2011) notes that the outcome of your study should be important and not trivial. Include outcomes that might be meaningful to the people who make decisions about healthcare practice. For example, suppose you researched whether adults who received supplemental feedings have an improved outcome of gaining weight. You would ask the question, "Do fragile geriatric individuals aged 65 and older gain weight when provided with supplemental calorie shakes with meals?" Your outcome for this intervention would be *gaining weight*. By specifically stating your outcome in your question, you can more accurately focus the search for evidence in the literature. As a result, you would find more relevant studies than if you searched for *protein shakes* alone.

Other Recommended Steps

Time Frame

Fineout-Overholt and Johnston (2005) recommended adding a fifth element to the PICOT method. The last component, "T," in the expanded PICOT acronym stands for time—the time frame in which the question occurs. While it is helpful to establish a timeline for completion of the PICOT process, parts of the process may be out of your control. Still, establishing deadlines helps you stay focused and on task.

Environment and Stakeholders

Schlosser, Koul, and Costello (2007) have proposed another approach, which they call the **PESICO** method. The acronym **stands for person, environment, stakeholders, intervention, comparison, and outcome**. These authors believe that environment should be included as a component of the research method, as it can directly affect the outcome, and that one must establish which of the stakeholders in a study stand to gain or lose. These important sources of influence need to be considered when undertaking an EBP project.

EVALUATING VALIDITY AND RELIABILITY

When examining research studies, **consider whether the study is reliable and valid**. These two terms should be understood and applied to your EBP project.

- **Validity** is the ability to measure what is supposed to or is intended to be measured.
- **Reliability** is the ability to measure what you want to measure on subsequent experiences.

Consider the following example. If your institution is purchasing new blood glucose meters, the meters should be tested to ensure that they accurately measure blood glucose levels every time (validity). The meters should also measure a blood glucose level of 100 the same way each time this test is performed on a patient (reliability). **To be valid and reliable, the meters should consistently meet these criteria.** (The need for valid and reliable equipment in the clinical environment is essential to safe practice and underscores why any nonfunctional piece of equipment should be removed immediately from service.) These terms will be explored in more detail in Chapter 7, Finding the Evidence.

The five cases that follow are designed to help define and focus your clinical question using the PICOT method.

CASE STUDIES

CASE STUDY 2.1

You work in a pediatric unit at a local hospital. Children are being read-mitted for rotavirus infection, which causes gastrointestinal illness that results in severe diarrhea and abdominal cramping. Children with this infection frequently present with severe dehydration. The virus is trans-mitted through contact by the fecal–oral route. Each of the readmitted chil-dren was in the hospital a week before this second admission for another illness. As you think about this, you realize that these children must be getting this infection nosocomially. You suspect handwashing may be a problem on your unit. You want to explore this occurrence through an EBP study. Fill in the blanks for the potential question of interest.

Does the incidence of readmission of pediatric patients younger than 8 years of age (P) decrease when proper handwashing/sanitizing is used by all healthcare personnel (I) as compared to not washing their hands (C) increase or decrease the readmission of patients (O) over the winter months from October to March (T)?

P = *pediatric patients younger than 8 years of age*
I = *adherence to hand sanitizing protocols*
C = *healthcare personnel washing/sanitizing their hands versus not washing/sanitizing hands*
O = *increase (or decrease) in the readmission of patients*
T = *over the winter months from October to March is more specific a time frame to examine*

CASE STUDY 2.2

You work in a busy ED in a level-one trauma center. You notice an increase in the number of young adult patients admitted with severe head injury. Your state has just changed the law so that motorcycle rid-ers are not required to wear helmets. Fill in the blanks here.

For patients younger than 25 years of age (P) does wearing a helmet (implied I) versus not wearing a helmet while riding a motorcycle (C) decrease the number of admissions for severe head injury (O)?

P = *patients younger than 25 years of age*
I = *wearing a helmet*
C = *wearing a helmet or not wearing a helmet*
O = *decrease the admission of motorcycle riders for severe head injury*

Note: Not every question will have an intervention component (as in a meaning question) or a time component (when it is implied in another part of the question). In this question the time is implied since the state just changed the law.

CASE STUDY 2.3

A 78-year-old man is at the physician's office for a regular checkup. His blood pressure is 160/98 mmHg. His physical examination results are otherwise normal. He normally takes blood pressure medication. When asked if he has been taking his medication regularly, he says yes and mentions that he also takes a multivitamin and some "natural remedies." He lives alone and is independent in all of his activities of daily living. His daughter, who visits him weekly, is with him for the appointment.

You ask both of them if you can do anything to assist him in "remembering" to take his medication. You consult the literature and find out that 75% of elderly individuals living alone forget to take their medications on a daily basis.

For elderly individuals older than 70 years of age living alone (**P**) does placing their medications weekly in a medication box marked with the days of the week, times of the day (**I**) versus not placing the medications in a pill box (**C**) increase their compliance or adherence to taking their medications and maintaining a stable blood pressure (**O**) over a weeks time (**T**)?

P = elderly individuals older than 70 years of age
I = placing their medications in a marked bill box
C = placing medications in the pill box versus not placing them in a pill box
O = increase compliance or adherence to taking their medications and keeping a stable blood pressure
T = within a week's time? Could be a month, whatever you want to test

CASE STUDY 2.4

You work in a rural hospital in the labor and delivery department. Within the past 6 months, you notice that the new certified nurse anesthetist and physicians have started offering epidural anesthesia for all routine vaginal deliveries. You note that of the last 100 vaginal deliveries, 89 involved epidural anesthesia. You wonder if this is necessary or *presented as a choice to the mother. You decide to consult the literature, looking for evidence.*

*For laboring patients scheduled for a vaginal delivery (**P**) over the past 6 months (**T**) was epidural anesthesia (**I**) appropriate as compared to a natural delivery (**C**) method for women with a uncomplicated vaginal delivery (**O**)?*

P = *laboring patients scheduled for vaginal delivery*
I = *administering epidural anesthesia*
C = *epidural anesthesia versus natural delivery method*
O = *was it necessary or needed*
T = *over the last 6 months*

CASE STUDY 2.5

You work in an adult intensive care burn unit. You notice that standard protocol stipulates that tube feedings are usually not started until the 5th day after admission to the burn unit. You wonder why tube feedings are not started earlier and whether that increases or decreases the length of stay of patients in the burn unit. You also wonder if patients are getting the proper nutrition, as you know they are in a hypermetabolic state because of their injuries. What effect does this have on their weight and nutritional status? You consult the literature to find studies on the timing of feeding adult burn unit patients. The literature shows that tube feeding started in the first 24 hours of admission to the burn unit decreased the morbidity and length of stay in burn units across the country.

*In adult burn patients older than 18 years of age (**P**), does starting tube feedings (**I**) on day 1 versus day 5 (**C**) of admission increase or decrease the length of stay (**O**) of patients in the burn unit?*

P = *adult burn patients older than 18 years of age in the burn unit*
I = *tube feedings*
C = *starting the feedings on day 1 or day 5*
O = *increase or decrease their length of stay*
T = *length of stay (you could be specific or not; measure it in days, weeks, or months)*

For this example you could also do a comparison of weight gain. Does starting tube feedings on day 1 versus day 5 alter the weight of an adult burn patient over 18 years of age admitted to the burn unit?

Fast Facts

Once you select a topic for your EBP project, be specific in defining your patient population and environment. If your question is too broad, it may not be answerable or you may not find evidence on that particular subject. By narrowing your question and asking it in an answerable format, you will increase the ease of developing your EBP project. A key is to see how well your question fits into an EBP model, such as the PICOT format.

REFERENCES

Adams, S. (2009). Identifying research questions. In N. A. Schmidt & J. M. Brown (Eds.), *Evidence-based practice for nurses: Appraisal and application of research* (pp. 57–74). Boston, MA: Jones & Bartlett.

Fineout-Overholt, E., & Johnston, L. (2005). Teaching EBP: Asking searchable, answerable clinical questions. *Worldviews on Evidence-Based Nursing, 2*(3), 157–160. doi:10.1111/j.1741-6787.2005.00032.x

Higgins, J. P. T., & Green, S. (2011, March) Cochrane handbook for systematic reviews of interventions (Version 5.1.0). Retrieved from http://community.cochrane.org/handbook

Melnyk, B. M., & Fineout-Overholt, E. (2010). *Evidence-based practice in nursing & healthcare: A guide to best practice* (2nd ed.). Philadelphia, PA: Lippincott Williams & Wilkins.

Sackett, D., Straus, S., Richardson, W., Rosenberg, W., & Hayes, R. (Eds.). (2000). *Evidence-based medicine: How to practice and teach EBM* (2nd ed.). New York, NY: Churchill Livingstone.

Schlosser, R. W., Koul, R., & Costello, J. (2007). Asking well-built questions for evidence-based practice in augmentative and alternative communication. *Journal of Communication Disorders, 40*(3), 225–238. doi:10.1016/j.jcomdis.2006.06.008

3

The Iowa Model of Evidence-Based Practice to Promote Quality Care

Evidence-based practice (EBP) improves the quality of patient care and clinical practice. Nurses need to use up-to-date research to deliver that care. The Iowa Model was designed with the idea that in order to choose a topic for an EBP project, either a knowledge-based or a problem-based trigger must be used. This model is used by many hospitals. This chapter explains this model.

In this chapter, you will:

1. Understand the history of the Iowa Model.
2. Review the steps of the Iowa Model.
3. Learn how to select a topic using a knowledge-based or a problem-based trigger.
4. Determine if the topic is a priority.
5. Formulate the EBP question and project.
6. Learn how to design and implement practice change.

INTRODUCTION TO THE IOWA MODEL OF EBP

The Iowa Model is a model of EBP and has been widely used and shared in academic and clinical settings. Since the original publication of this model by Titler et al. in 1994, the authors have received many written requests to use the model in publications and presentations. The

The Iowa Model focuses on **problem-focused triggers** or **knowledge-based triggers**. Problem-focused triggers come from issues identified by staff as problems. Knowledge-based triggers are generated when staff members read nursing or research journals or attend a conference and reflect on a topic and seek to understand.

Iowa Model was developed by a team of nurses from the University of Iowa Hospitals and Clinics, and the College of Nursing developed this framework that was originally called the Iowa Model of Research-Based Practice to Promote Quality Care (Figure 3.1), to guide clinicians in evaluating and using research findings in patient care (Iowa Model Collaborative, 2017). Many hospital systems are using this model as the basis for their EBP initiatives. The authors of the Iowa Model adopted the definition of EBP as a thoughtful and careful use of current best evidence to guide healthcare decisions. In the Iowa Model evidence ranges from meta-analysis to case reports and expert opinions. In this model either knowledge-focused or problem-focused "triggers" are what lead staff members to look at and question current nursing practice and determine if patient care can be improved using research findings. The steps in the Iowa Model process are as follows:

1. Select a topic.
2. Form a team.
3. Retrieve evidence.
4. Grade the evidence.
5. Develop an EBP standard.
6. Implement the EBP.
7. Evaluate the EBP.

Now let's look at the process. The first thing is to select a topic. Sounds easy, but many of the graduates who are new to the unit, and for whom this is a component of their nurse residency program, must complete an EBP project. They have no idea where to start or how to come up with an idea. They are too inexperienced to know current practice problems, so they rely on the wisdom of their senior staff or clinical educator. While that is fine, it is very important that the new graduates have an interest in the topic. The graduates can choose the topic but should get approval from their unit or clinical educator in charge of EBP projects. So the simple thing a new graduate can do is to "listen" and "wonder why." Listen to what staff, patients, physicians, and others are saying is problematic in the unit. This could be a great way to come up with an idea. Ask peers if they think it is feasible and if it has been looked at before. The other thing is to wonder why we do things in a certain way. Yours are a new set of eyes. You should question everything when you are new. Always ask why. If the answer does not make sense, look for some evidence. Then, depending on what you find, determine if this might be a good EBP project. Many new graduates find selecting the topic as the hardest part.

Selecting a Topic

Problem-focused triggers come from issues identified by staff as problems, issues identified through quality improvement initiatives or audits, as a result of risk management surveillance, incident reports, patient safety events, or recurring clinical problems. For example, why do postoperative patients wind up with a deep vein thrombus? **Knowledge-based triggers** are generated when staff members read nursing or research journals or attend a conference and reflect on a topic and seek to understand. For example, you may read a journal article on placement of postpyloric feeding tubes and look at the evidence and the process you use in the unit you work and see whether your unit is following the latest recommendations. Some ideas put forth by LoBiondo-Wood and Haber (2014) that can be used as selection criteria for an EBP project are as follows:

1. The priority of the topic for nursing and the organization
2. The magnitude of the problem (large, moderate, or small)
3. Applicability to several or a few clinical areas
4. The likelihood of the change to improve the quality of care, decrease length of stay, contain costs, or improve patient satisfaction
5. Potential "landmines" associated with the topic and the capability to diffuse them
6. Availability of baseline quality improvement or risk data that will be helpful during evaluation
7. Multidisciplinary nature of the topic and the ability to create collaborative relationships to effect the needed changes
8. Interest and commitment of staff to the potential topic
9. Availability of a sound body of evidence, preferably research evidence

These nine triggers were then simplified in 2015 into five triggers, which combine problem-based and knowledge-based triggers. They are:

1. Clinical or patient-identified issues*
2. Organizational, state, or national initiatives
3. Data/new evidence

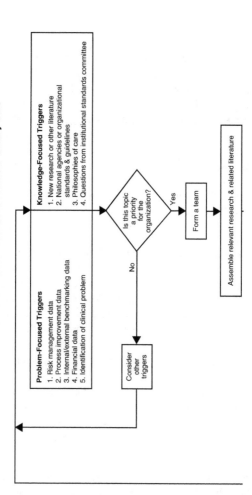

The Iowa Model of
Evidence-Based Practice to Promote Quality Care

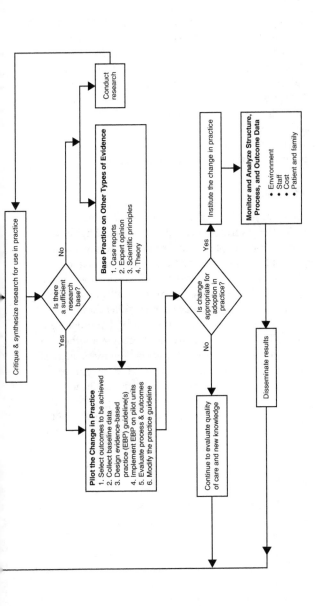

Figure 3.1 The Iowa Model of Research-Based Practice to Promote Quality Care.
Source: Reprinted with permission from the University of Iowa Hospitals and Clinics, Copyright 1998.

Chapter **3** **The Iowa Model of Evidence-Based Practice to Promote Quality Care**

4. Accrediting agency requirements or regulations*
5. Philosophy of care

As a result of a study of 431 participants who requested to access the Iowa Model from 2001 to 2013, 88 percent ($n = 379$) identified problematic steps when using the model. These steps were topic priority, critique, pilot, and institute change. As a result changes were made to the model. The revised model is explained in this chapter. As described earlier the nine original triggers were consolidated into five. A step was added to the model to state the question or purpose of the EBP project. Formally stating the purpose would allow a more focused approach to synthesize the body of evidence to decide if the topic is a priority. All of this information is illustrated in Figure 3.2 (Iowa Model Collaborative, 2017).

Is This Topic a Priority?

This is an important point in that if the topic chosen is not a priority or in line with the institution's mission or vision or not linked to the organization's strategic plan, it is unlikely to receive resources and backing to implement it into practice. If the topic is not a priority, the model suggests choosing another topic (Iowa Model Collaborative, 2017). Remember what the deciding point was in choosing your topic: Is it to implement practice change? What do you hope to accomplish? If a topic is chosen just for the sake of it, it probably will not be worth the effort, and it would be wise to choose another topic. Also, to know if your topic is a priority, ask yourself these questions: Is this topic relevant to the patient's preferences for care and/or quality of life? Is there an economic burden associated with the topic (loss of work, etc.)? Would it improve a process in your practice setting? Would it improve safety for the patient, family, or staff? Are there any new-evidence data that should drive a change in practice? Would it enable a way for innovation in practice? (Cullen et al., 2018).

Forming a Team

Choosing who will be on your team is crucial to the success of the project. This team will be responsible for the development, implementation, and evaluation of your project. Be sure the team is all on board with the topic selected. This team can be a unit-based committee or a freely formed new group of people. It can be interdisciplinary, depending on the topic chosen. To develop EBP at unit level, the team should draw up written policies, procedures, and guidelines that are evidence based (LoBiondo-Wood & Haber, 2014). Discussion

---

* Newly added.

should take place between the organization's direct care providers and leadership such as nurse managers to support these changes. Failure to involve stakeholders and leadership in this process may cause the EBP initiative to fail. Also remember the team may change over time. Think about the skill sets needed to plan, conduct, and implement the project. Important activities and qualities of the team are reviewing the literature, obtaining baseline data, and engaging key stakeholders (Iowa Model Collaborative, 2017). Also, not all team members need to be involved in every aspect of the project. For example, if you need someone from the IT (information technology) team to help you gather data, that person would not necessarily be needed to assist with review of the literature. Or the librarian who assists you in finding the literature may not be needed to work on other aspects of the project. The team should be fluent and serve a purpose. This purpose can be brief or could be long term.

Formulate the EBP Question

Another important task of the EBP team is to formulate the EBP question. What is it you want to know? This will help set boundaries around the project and keep it focused. A clearly defined question should involve people/patients, interventions or exposures, outcomes, and relevant study designs (Alderson, Green, & Higgins, 2004). There are many ways to formulate the question. One method, summarized in Table 3.1, is the PICOT (patient or population, intervention, comparison, outcome, time) method by Melynyk and Fineout-Overholt (see Chapter 2, Asking the Compelling Question). A clearly defined question is vital to the success of the project. Clearly identify what types of people/patients are going to be examined, what intervention might be used, and what outcomes are expected. Stillwell, Fineout-Overholt, Melnyk, and Williamson (2010) describe two types of questions. **Background questions** are broad and provide general knowledge. They usually begin with *when* or *what*, for example: What is the best way to take a temperature in children? What is compassion fatigue? When do the effects of ketamine wear off? The other type of question is a **foreground question**. This type of question is so specific that when answered it provides evidence for clinical decision making. A foreground question may follow the PICOT method (see Chapter 2, Asking the Compelling Question; Stillwell et al., 2010).

EXAMPLES

In a critically injured trauma patient (P—patient population of interest), does feeding them early (I—intervention) versus not feeding

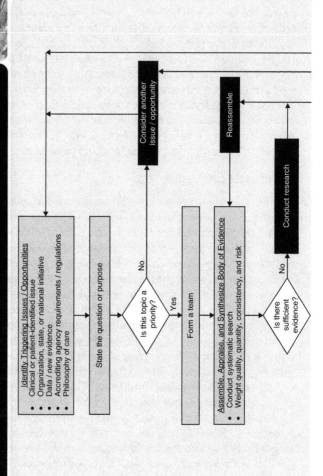

The Iowa Model Revised : Evidence-Based Practice to Promote Excellence in Health Care

Identify Triggering Issues / Opportunities
- Clinical or patient-identified issue
- Organization, state, or national initiative
- Data / new evidence
- Accrediting agency requirements / regulations
- Philosophy of care

State the question or purpose

Is this topic a priority?

No → Consider another issue / opportunity

Yes → Form a team

Assemble, Appraise, and Synthesize Body of Evidence
- Conduct systematic search
- Weight quality, quantity, consistency, and risk

Is there sufficient evidence?

No → Conduct research

Reassemble

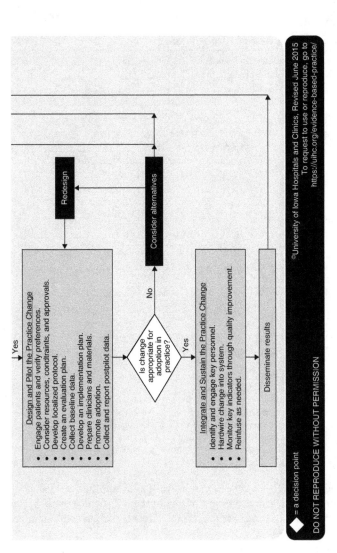

Yes

Design and Pilot the Practice Change
• Engage patients and verify preferences.
• Consider resources, constraints, and approvals.
• Develop localized protocol.
• Create an evaluation plan.
• Collect baseline data.
• Develop an implementation plan.
• Prepare clinicians and materials.
• Promote adoption.
• Collect and report postpilot data.

Redesign

Consider alternatives

No

Is change appropriate for adoption in practice?

Yes

Integrate and Sustain the Practice Change
• Identify and engage key personnel.
• Hardwire change into system.
• Monitor key indicators through quality improvement.
• Reinfuse as needed.

Disseminate results

◆ = a decision point

DO NOT REPRODUCE WITHOUT PERMISSION

©University of Iowa Hospitals and Clinics, Revised June 2015
To request to use or reproduce, go to
https://uihc.org/evidence-based-practice/

Figure 3.2 The Iowa Model—Revised.
Source: Reprinted with permission from the University of Iowa Hospitals and Clinics, Copyright 2015.

Chapter **3** The Iowa Model of Evidence-Based Practice to Promote Quality Care

Table 3.1

Templates and Definitions for PICOT Questions

Question Type	Definition	Template
Intervention or therapy	To determine which treatment leads to the best outcome	In _____(P), how does _____(I) compared with _____(C) affect _____(O) within _____(T)?
Etiology	To determine the greatest risk factors or causes of a condition	Are _____(P) who have _____(I), compared with those without _____(C), at _____risk for _____(O) over _____(T)?
Diagnosis or diagnostic test	To determine which test is more accurate and precise in diagnosing a condition	In _____(P), are/is _____(I) compared with _____(C) more accurate in diagnosing _____(O)?
Prognosis or prediction	To determine the clinical course over time and likely complications of a condition	In _____(P), how does _____(I) compared with _____(C), influence _____(O) over _____(T)?
Meaning	To understand the meaning of an experience for a particular individual, group, or community	How do _____(P) with _____(I) perceive _____(O) during _____(T)?

PICOT, patient or population, intervention, comparison, outcome, time.
Source: Stillwell, S., Fineout-Overholt, E., Melnyk, B., & Williamson, K. (2010). Evidence-based practice: Step by step: Asking the clinical question. A key step in evidence-based practice. *American Journal of Nursing, 110*(3), 58–61. doi:10.1097/01. NAJ.0000368959.11129.79

them early (C—comparison of interest) affect morbidity (O—outcome of interest) and length of stay in the ICU (which could be a second O—outcome of interest or T—time it takes to demonstrate the outcome)?

In hospitalized patients (P), does hourly rounding (I) versus rounding every 4 hours (C) affect fall rates (O) in medical-surgical units?

In infants younger than 1 year of age (P), does keeping side rails all the way up (I) decrease fall rates (C) versus having the crib rails half way up (O)?

As proposed by Stillwell et al. (2010), the preceding are some of the different question types. You can then decide if you would like to investigate an intervention or therapy, an etiology or cause, a diagnosis or diagnostic test, or a prediction or prognosis over time or to understand the meaning or experience for a particular group of individuals (see Table 3.1).

Assemble, Appraise, and Synthesize the Body of Evidence

This used to be a two-step process in the old model. The new Iowa Model suggests that evidence be grouped to emphasize the entire body of literature, not just the research studies (Iowa Model Collaborative, 2017). (Please see Chapter 8, Evaluating the Evidence.)

Is There Sufficient Evidence?

There is some struggle in determining what is "enough" evidence and what is sufficient. Include multiple types of evidence. Before recommending a practice change, be sure to base your decisions using the strongest of the evidence. Always remember practice should *never* be changed based on one research study or one piece of evidence. There may not be any evidence at all. Perhaps that is why you chose the topic; do consider conducting a research study. There are resources in almost every institution that can guide you in this process. Again what is important is to get buy-in by the key stakeholders. For example, if you are looking at a practice change in the hospital, it is important to have nursing, physician, and administrative buy-in prior to conducting a research study. If you get buy-in, these stakeholders should be on the research team.

Design and Pilot the Practice Change

One big change from the previous model was to make this revised model patient focused versus institution focused. Also, there was a need to address necessary resources (do you have enough committee participants to carry out the project), constraints by administration, leadership, and supporting team members. There are also approvals required for example if there is a potential to harm; the human subjects committee or institutional review board (IRB) approval may be needed. Approval is also needed by the institution's division of education to organize and maintain consistency in process and implementation. Someone needs to be in charge of overseeing all the EBP projects in the institution. Look at whatever time constraints and approvals may be needed in the road ahead to implement the practice change. Another important aspect to change is to look at current practice protocols and determine if they are specific to a particular unit or setting or if they may require further modifications when attempting to apply them elsewhere (in other units, settings, or patient population; Iowa Model Collaborative, 2017).

- Engage patients and verify preferences.
- Consider resources, constraints, and approval.
- Develop localized protocol.
- Create an evaluation plan.
- Collect baseline data.
- Develop an implementation plan.
- Prepare clinicians and materials.
- Promote adoption.
- Collect and report postpilot data.

Is the Change Appropriate for Adoption?

This next decision point on the Iowa Model of EBP is to decide if the change is appropriate for adoption into practice. If the answer is yes, then adopt it. If the answer is no, then one would want to reconsider any alternatives and a potential redesign to the project. For example, if the findings do not match those anticipated from the evidence, then the team needs to consider alternatives to the practice change or revise the implantation plan (Iowa Model Collaborative, 2017).

Integrate and Sustain the Practice Change

This may be the most difficult step, as implementing change always is. How does one make change sustainable? A suggestion is to show the linkage with quality improvement methods, as a foundational step for sustaining change—that is, by implementing a quality improvement process, it will provide a foundation to not only initiate change but also for that change to be maintained and be sustainable in the future (Rocker & Verma, 2014). Other components are to:

- Identify and engage key personnel.
- Hardwire change into the system.
- Monitor key indicators through quality improvement initiatives.
- Reinfuse as needed (and re-excite personnel).

In the integration phase, identifying and engaging key personnel is crucial to success, even if this requires forming a new team and identifying new champions of the initiative. Hardwiring change means to embed the new practice into the organization. Also it is vital to monitor through the quality improvement/performance improvement committees if the changes made actually improved practice. Then, as always, reinfuse the energy (Iowa Model Collaborative, 2017). You need to be the cheerleader and keep people excited about the project and change. How are things better now? More important, how did the practice change impact patients and patient care for the good?

Disseminate Your Results

If you have found your EBP project to be useful and impact practice in a positive way, share it with the world. Disseminate the results. Definitely share it with the rest of your institution, but also consider publishing or presenting (by poster or a podium presentation) the results at local, national, and international conferences. There are journals devoted strictly to EBP initiatives. But do not keep the information to yourself; share it and help others.

CONCLUSION

In conclusion, this chapter familiarizes you with the Iowa Model of EBP. Updates were made to the prior model because of a research study that was conducted by a team of nurses. Information about both the previous and current models is shared in this chapter.

REFERENCES

Alderson, P., Green, S., & Higgins, J. (2004). *Cochrane Reviewers Handbook 4.2.1.* Retrieved from https://www.iecs.org.ar/cochrane/guias/Handbook_4-2-2.pdf

Cullen, L., Hanrahan, K., Farrington, M., DeBerg, J., Tucker, S., & Kleiber, C. (2018). *Evidence-based practice in action: Comprehensive strategies, tools, and tips from the University of Iowa Hospitals and Clinics.* Indianapolis, IN: Sigma Theta Tau International.

Iowa Model Collaborative. (2017). Iowa model of evidence-based practice: Revisions and validation. *Worldviews on Evidence-Based Nursing, 14*(3), 175–182. doi:10.1111/wvn.12223

LoBiondo-Wood, G., & Haber, J. (2014). *Nursing research: Methods and critical appraisal for evidence based practice* (8th ed.). St. Louis, MO: Mosby.

Rocker, G. M., & Verma, J. Y. (2014). "INSPIRED" COPD outreach program™: Doing the right things right. *Clinical and Investigative Medicine, 37*(5), E311–E319. doi:10.25011/cim.v37i5.22011

Stillwell, S., Fineout-Overholt, E., Melnyk, B., & Williamson, K. (2010). Evidence-based practice: Step by step: Asking the clinical question. A key step in evidence-based practice. *American Journal of Nursing, 110*(3), 58–61. doi:10.1097/01.NAJ.0000368959.11129.79

Titler, M. G., Kleiber, C., Steelman, V., Goode, C., Rakel, B., Barry-Walker, J.,... Buckwalter, K. (1994). Infusing research into practice to promote quality care. *Nursing Research, 43*(5), 307–313. Retrieved from http://www.ncbi.nlm.nih.gov/pubmed/7937178

4

A Basic Understanding of Research

You might think that now that you have decided on a compelling question, you are ready to search for evidence. But before beginning your evidence-based practice (EBP) project, you need to understand some basic principles. That way, when you find evidence, you will know what type it is, how to classify and interpret it, and whether the research finding constitutes "good evidence." This chapter provides an overview of the research process as well as the proper terminology. For additional explanations about the process, consult a research text. Remember that you will not be conducting a research study. Rather, you will be conducting an EBP project.

In this chapter, you will learn:

1. A basic history of nursing research
2. The two basic types of research
3. The steps in the research process

A HISTORY OF NURSING RESEARCH

When did nursing research begin? Florence Nightingale introduced the concept of scientific inquiry as the basis of nursing practice. She began collecting information and making observations about soldier mortality and morbidity during the Crimean War. With these scientific data, she fought for changes in nursing practice that affected outcomes for soldiers in the war (Houser, 2008). Her work to improve sanitary conditions in the 1800s was one of the first times a nurse linked environmental conditions (variables) to clinical or patient outcomes. Nightingale also kept detailed notes on her patients. Her book *Notes on Nursing* presents her initial observations and findings. **Although Nightingale did not practice evidence-based research, her findings were based on her experience and observations.** Although simplistic by today's methods, her approach reflects a rudimentary form of the nursing research process.

TWO BASIC CATEGORIES OF RESEARCH

The two **main categories of nursing research are quantitative and qualitative**. In quantitative studies, the researcher identifies variables of interest and collects relevant data from subjects. These data usually take on a numerical format (Polit & Beck, 2016). For example, suppose the researcher is measuring happiness using a quantitative approach. The researcher would need to quantify happiness using a numerical happiness scale on which subjects could objectively quantify their level of happiness. An example would be a scale of 0 to 10 on a continuum, where 0 is no happiness and 10 is extreme happiness.

In qualitative studies, the researcher collects narrative data or descriptions by having conversations with the research participants, making observations, and taking notes. These interactions usually occur in the participants' natural environments, such as home, workplace, or a mutually agreed upon venue. Diaries may also be used (Polit & Beck, 2016). If the preceding happiness study was a qualitative study, the researcher would ask participants to describe their happiness by using a broad inquiry, such as "Tell me about your happiness," and paying careful attention not to persuade or influence the participants' answers.

Table 4.1 compares data obtained from qualitative and quantitative research approaches in a study on pain. These research methods are discussed in greater depth in Chapter 5, Quantitative Research, and Chapter 6, Qualitative Research.

Table 4.1

Example of Quantitative Data Versus Qualitative Data: Pain	
Quantitative Study	**Qualitative Study**
Numerical scale, 0 to 10	Verbal description, "Tell me more about your pain"
"The pain was 3 out of 10"	"The pain was crushing and the worst I ever had"

Quantitative Research

Quantitative research is objective. It imposes tight control over the research situation. It generalizes findings and frequently includes numbers, facts, and figures (see Chapter 5, Quantitative Research). When you think of quantitative research, think **numbers**. The study sample usually has a large number of participants or subjects.

Qualitative Research

Qualitative research is more subjective. It describes an individual's experience in the his or her own words. This narrative or verbal description is obtained after the researcher asks the participant an open-ended question and allows the participant to share his or her thoughts and feelings (see Chapter 5, Quantitative Research). Qualitative research usually has fewer participants in the sample than those with quantitative studies. Statistical analysis is used, and common themes are sought and identified. For further clarification of this analysis, consult a basic research text.

Fast Facts

- Quantitative research is objective.
- Qualitative research is subjective.

STEPS IN THE RESEARCH PROCESS

The steps in the research process are summarized in Box 4.1 and described in the pages that follow. Some steps may overlap, some can be varied, and some can be combined.

Step One: Identify the Problem (Problem Statement)

The first and perhaps **the most important part of the research process is to clearly identify the problem.** What is it that the researcher wants to study? This problem should be of interest to the researcher and should also be of significance to nursing. For example, a pediatric nurse may be interested in studying the best method of measuring temperature in a child, but the question is whether the conclusion would really make a difference to the field of nursing. A review of the literature reveals that this topic has been studied frequently, with 35 studies agreeing on the most accurate method. This topic clearly does not need to be studied again. Now, suppose that same nurse learns that a new

BOX 4.1   STEPS IN THE RESEARCH PROCESS

1. Identify the problem.
2. State the purpose of the study.
3. Determine the study variables.
4. Conduct a review of the literature.
5. Identify a theoretical or conceptual framework.
6. Conduct the study ethically.
7. Identify study assumptions.
8. Formulate the hypothesis or research questions.
9. Identify the type of research design.

device for temperature taking, such as a femoral thermometer, has just been invented. If the nurse wants to study whether the femoral method is as accurate as the rectal method, this is a new and important question. By conducting this research study, one could determine if this new method is indeed accurate and, if so, if it should be recommended as the preferred method for use in pediatric units across the country.

The problem statement can be one declarative or interrogative sentence that includes a clear identification of the population to be studied and the variables involved. The last thing for the researcher to consider is whether the problem is empirically testable. The problem statement is the "what" of the study. What is going to be examined by the researcher, and can it be done?

Fast Facts

Declarative statement: *Femoral thermometer readings are more accurate than those obtained with the rectal method in pediatric patients from 1 to 4 years of age.*

Interrogative statement: *Are femoral thermometers as accurate as rectal thermometers in pediatric patients from 1 to 4 years of age?*

There are many things to consider when writing a good problem statement. See Box 4.2 for guidelines in writing and critiquing the problem statement.

Step Two: State the Purpose of the Study

This step defines the reason for the study. What is the purpose? **Why does one want to study this topic?** What is the goal, or aim?

BOX 4.2 GUIDELINES FOR WRITING AND CRITIQUING A PROBLEM STATEMENT

- Is the problem statement clear and concise?
- Is the problem statement written as a declarative or an interrogatory sentence?
- Are the study variables and population of interest included in the problem statement?
- Does the problem statement indicate that the study would be feasible or able to be carried out?
- Does the problem statement indicate that it is clinically significant or relevant to nursing practice?

Source: Adapted from Nieswiadomy, R. M. (2012). *Foundations of nursing research* (6th ed.). Upper Saddle River, NJ: Pearson.

For example, the statement of purpose for the problem identified earlier, which involves methods of measuring temperature in pediatric patients, might read as follows: "The purpose of the study is to determine which method of measuring temperature in pediatric patients from 1 to 4 years of age is more accurate." Sometimes the problem statement and the purpose are seen as the same, but they really are not. The problem statement is the "what" of the study. It formally identifies the problem being addressed. It includes the scope of the research problem, the specific population being studied, the independent and dependent variables, and the goal or question the study is trying to answer (Gillis & Jackson, 2002). In comparison, the purpose of the study is the "why" of what is being examined, and it derives from the problem statement (Adams, 2009). Both statements should be mentioned near the beginning of the study.

Fast Facts

Problem statements identify "what" the study is about; the purpose statement identifies "why" the study is being conducted.

Step Three: Determine the Study Variables

In an experimental study, the concepts or items of interest to be studied are called variables. A variable is something that can change. For example, weight, age, and body temperature are all variables that can be studied (Polit & Beck, 2016). **Variables can be independent**

or dependent. An independent variable is the "cause," or the variable that influences the dependent variable. The **dependent variable** is the "effect," or that which is influenced by the independent variable. The dependent variable can also be called the **criterion** or **outcome variable**. It is the variable that is observed for change or reaction after the intervention has been applied (Fain, 2009). The reason for this is that in experimental research, researchers actively introduce an intervention or treatment to address therapy questions. In nonexperimental research, the researchers are bystanders; they collect data without making changes or introducing treatments (Polit & Beck, 2016). For examples of independent and dependent variables, see Box 4.3.

For example, if the researcher was looking at the relationship between age and the amount of exercise people engage in, the independent variable would be age, and the dependent variable would be exercise. In this case, age is not the cause of the amount of exercise performed, but it is the direction of influence on the item or issue identified that influences the second variable (exercise; Nieswiadomy, 2012). It is clear from this example that age may have a direct influence on the amount of exercise a person is able to do. So, this is another way that variables play an important role in the research process. For more on variables, see Chapter 5, Quantitative Research.

What, indeed, are the variables included in a study? There may be one, two, or many variables in a study. A one-variable study is also called a **univariate study**. An example of a problem statement

BOX 4.3 EXAMPLES OF INDEPENDENT AND DEPENDENT VARIABLES

- In the hospital, does the presence of a support group for head-injured patients affect the stress level of patients with head injuries?

    Independent variable (IV) = presence of support group;
    Dependent variable (DV) = stress level of patients

- Is there a difference between the development of breast cancer in women who eat meat and those who do not eat meat?

    IV = those who eat meat and do not eat meat;
    DV = development of breast cancer

- Is there a difference in NCLEX® test scores between baccalaureate nursing (BSN) students and associate degree nursing (ADN) students?

    IV = BSN students and ADN students;
    DV = test scores

with only one variable would be "What are the sources of stress in the emergency department?" Here the researcher is only looking at one variable as the source of stress.

A two-variable study is also called a **bivariate study**. Usually, one variable is the independent variable, and the second, a dependent variable. An example of a bivariate study question is "Does the speed of driving correlate to the incidence of automobile accidents in adolescents?" An automobile accident is the independent variable, and the speed of the car is the dependent variable. A second example of a bivariate study question is the following interrogatory problem statement: "Does the level of stress affect final exam scores for senior BSN students?" The cause or level of stress in this case will have a direct effect on the final exam scores, which is the dependent variable. Table 4.2 offers examples of types of problem statements using variables.

Fast Facts

An independent variable is the "cause," or the variable that influences the dependent variable. The dependent variable is the "effect," or that which is influenced by the independent variable.

Table 4.2

Variables in Problem Statement Format

Correlational statement	Is there a correlation between X (independent variable) and Y (the dependent variable)? *Example: Is there a correlation between the level of stress and final exam scores of nursing students?*
Comparative statement	Is there a difference in Y (dependent variable) between people who have X (independent variable) and those who do not have X? *Example: Is there a difference in stress levels of nursing students who had a review course and those who did not have a review course?*
Experimental study statement	Is there a difference in Y (dependent variable) between a group that received X (independent variable) and those who did not receive X (independent variable)? *Example: Is there a difference in pain in pediatric patients who received EMLA cream and those who did not receive EMLA cream prior to venipuncture?*

EMLA, Eutectic Mixture of Local Anesthetics.

There are other types of variables. **Extraneous variables**, for example, are those that are not under investigation or examination but still may (or may not) be relevant to, or interfere with, the study. Extraneous variables may be controlled or uncontrolled by the researcher. It is best for the researcher to try to identify any extraneous variables and control them so that they will not interfere with the purpose of the experiment or result in any adverse or unplanned effects. Extraneous variables may also be called **confounding variables**, **intervening variables**, or **mediating variables** (Fain, 2009; LoBiondo-Wood & Haber, 2014). An example of an extraneous variable occurs in the study of older men who are enrolled in a new exercise program (independent variable) to determine how exercise affects their lung condition (dependent variable) by measuring functional lung capacity. The extraneous variables that could affect the dependent variable would be age, a history of smoking (including the length of time and the amount the patient smoked), secondhand smoke exposure, and comorbid conditions, such as chronic obstructive pulmonary disease (COPD), lung cancer, asthma, or any diagnosis that might affect the dependent variable of actual functional lung capacity. So, the researcher would be wise to address these issues by eliminating from the study men who had smoked and had a preexisting or comorbid condition of COPD and asthma.

Step Four: Conduct a Review of the Literature

The review of the literature can be an overwhelming task for the novice researcher. If you are having difficulty conducting the literature review, consult a colleague or a librarian who is experienced with the process of finding research articles. They are excellent resources and usually are willing to help.

Research in any field must build on what already has been done. Therefore, **nurse researchers must locate relevant studies about the problem of interest to determine where the gaps in the literature are** and what areas need to be examined. Making yourself aware of relevant studies helps prevent duplication of what already has been done. Chapter 8, Evaluating the Evidence, provides guidelines for conducting the literature review.

Another skill is learning how to identify good literature and research. This process also allows the researcher to discover what instruments or tools have been used to study the topic of interest as well as the conceptual or theoretical frameworks applied. In the case of EBP, it also enables the researcher to determine if the evidence available advises a change in practice. Some questions may reveal a lack of evidence or research on a given topic. This should alert the researcher to the need for further research on the topic of interest.

Often, researchers ask how far back in the literature they should search. Generally, the researcher should look for relevant studies or literature within the past 5 years. However, if no research has been published within this time frame, the researcher will need to go back further. In either case, it is always appropriate to include landmark studies, even if they are more than 5 years old. **Landmark studies** are those that are **paramount to the direction of study of the topic**.

Step Five: Identify a Theoretical or Conceptual Framework

Nursing research is not conducted just to learn the answer to a specific question or to test a hypothesis. When a study is placed in a theoretical context, it allows one to speculate on the questions of why and how treatments work and how variables relate to each other (Polit & Beck, 2016). **Theory provides the structure for a research study.** It allows the researcher to generalize beyond a specific situation and predict what should happen in similar situations (McEwen & Wills, 2002). Good research integrates findings into an orderly and coherent system. Meleis (2007) states that the goal of theory in research "is to formulate a minimum set of generalizations that allow one to explain a maximum number of observational relationships among the variables in a given field of inquiry" (p. 45). She further states that the relationship between theory and research is cyclical in nature. The result of research can be used to verify, modify, disprove, or support a theoretical proposition. Nursing theory has provided new propositions that would not have been articulated if theories from other disciplines were used. Nursing theory is, therefore, very important.

For example, if a research study was conducted for examining the level of comfort a patient experiences postoperatively without pain medications, the study could be guided by Kolcaba's comfort theory (2019) or Roy's adaptation model (Barone, Roy, & Frederickson, 2008).

The word *theory* can be used in many ways. Scientists use theory to mean an abstract generalization that offers a systematic explanation of how phenomena are interrelated (Polit & Beck, 2016). It can also be categorized as descriptive, which Fawcett (1999) defines as an empirically driven theory that can be used to "describe or classify specific dimensions or characteristics of individuals, groups, situations, or events by summarizing commonalities found in discrete observations" (p. 15).

A **metaparadigm is a primary phenomenon** that is of interest to a particular discipline (Fawcett, 1999). Within nursing, the primary or central phenomena are the concepts of person, environment, health, and nursing (Fain, 2009). The theories that deal with these four metaparadigm concepts are referred to as nursing theories.

There are also traditional nursing theories that differ in their level of generality. **Grand theories are complex and broad** in scope. They include many concepts that are not usually grounded in empirical data (i.e., data gathered through the senses using objective measurement) or evidence. Therefore, they are not very useful in creating guidelines for nursing practice (Fain, 2009). **Middle range theories focus on only one piece of reality or the human experience, but they involve a selected number of concepts** (e.g., theories of stress; Polit & Beck, 2016). **Practice theories are more targeted than middle range theories and produce specific directions or guidelines for practice.** An example is the theories of end-of-life decision making (Fain, 2009). **Prescriptive theories address nursing therapeutics and the outcomes of interventions.** A prescriptive theory includes propositions that call for change and predict the consequences of a certain strategy for nursing intervention (Meleis, 2007). **Borrowed theories are taken from another discipline**, for example, psychology, and applied to nursing questions and research problems (Fain, 2009). Box 4.4 lists several such theories from other disciplines.

The building blocks of theories are called concepts. These are "words or phrases that convey a unique idea or mental image that is relevant to the theory" (Schmidt & Brown, 2009, p. 106). In other words, they describe a phenomenon that is an aspect of reality that can be consciously observed, sensed, or experienced. Phenomena within a discipline such as nursing (e.g., caring) reflect that domain (caring for a patient in nursing as compared to caring about what one will eat for dinner; Meleis, 2007). As such, a concept gives some degree of classification or categorization (Meleis, 2007).

BOX 4.4 THEORIES FROM DISCIPLINES OTHER THAN NURSING

Child development theory (Piaget; Freud; Erickson)
Family systems theory (Bowen)
Motivational theory (Maslow)
Social learning theory (Bandura)
Stress theory (Selye)
Stress and coping theory (Selye; Lazarus & Folkman)

BOX 4.5   NURSING THEORIES

Nursing Theory
http://www.nursing-theory.org/

Current Nursing Theory
http://currentnursing.com/nursing_theory/nursing_theorists.html

Nursing Theory and Models
http://www.nursing-theory.org/theories-and-models/

Constructs are higher level concepts that are derived from theories and represent nonobservable behaviors (Fain, 2009). A conceptual model is the same as a conceptual framework, which is a set of abstract and general concepts assembled to address a phenomenon of central interest (Polit & Beck, 2016). It represents ideas or notions that have been assembled in a specific way to represent or describe a particular area of concern. Conceptual models are loosely constructed in comparison to theories (Fain, 2009).

So where does one find a nursing theory to use with a research study? See Box 4.5 for websites that provide information about nursing theories.

Step Six: Keep the Study Ethical

All studies should be conducted ethically. Questions to consider include the following: Were study participants subjected to any physical harm, discomfort, or psychological distress? Did the researchers take appropriate steps to remove them from harm? Did the benefits to participants outweigh any potential risks? Did the benefits to society outweigh the costs to the participants? Was any type of coercion or undue influence used in recruiting or selecting the participants? Were vulnerable subjects used? Were the participants deceived or tricked in any way? Were they fully aware of participating in a study, and did they understand the purpose of the research? Were appropriate consent procedures used? Were appropriate steps taken to safeguard the privacy of participants? Was the research approved and monitored by an institutional review board (IRB) or other similar ethics review committee? All of these things need to be considered when evaluating a research study.

Step Seven: Identify Study Assumptions

Assumptions are "statements and principles that are taken as truth, based on a person's values and beliefs" (Fain, 2009, p. 192).

Assumptions are presumed to be true but may not indeed have been proved. Nieswiadomy (2012) describes three types of assumptions:

1. Universal assumptions. An example would be that all humans need love.
2. Assumptions based on a theory or research findings. For example, a study based on the finding that worrying leads to stress must identify the assumption that worry leads to stress so that a study on stress can use this assumption as its basis.
3. Assumptions that are necessary to complete the study. For example, if someone is studying women who commit murder and the study is conducted in a prison ward with convicted female murderers, it can be assumed that the women did indeed commit murder. That is how assumptions work.

Every scientific study or investigation is based on assumptions. Therefore, the researcher should state these assumptions clearly so factors that may have influenced the questions asked and other parts of the study are identified.

Step Eight: Formulate the Hypothesis and/or Research Questions

The researcher's expected findings form his or her **hypothesis**. The hypothesis is what ultimately **predicts the relationship between two or more variables**. The problem statement asks the question of interest, and the hypothesis then predicts the answer. The hypothesis should contain the population of interest and the variables, just as the problem statement does. A hypothesis must be able to be tested in a real-life situation (Nieswiadomy, 2012). Remember that the independent variable is the "cause," and the dependent variable is the "effect." There are several types of hypotheses, but only a few are discussed here.

A **research hypothesis** is a statement that shows an expected relationship between the variables. A **null hypothesis**, on the other hand, shows a complete lack of or absence of relationship between the variables (Polit & Beck, 2016). The null hypothesis is important when looking at statistics related to a study.

The directional type of research hypothesis is preferred for nursing studies (Nieswiadomy, 2012). A **directional hypothesis** shows that a relationship exists between the variables but that there is also an expected direction to that relationship. For example:

- There is a relationship between increased smoking and the increased risk of acquiring lung cancer. *(An obvious positive relationship is shown: increased smoking and increased risk of acquiring lung cancer.)*

- Older people are more susceptible to motor vehicle accidents because their reflexes are slower than those of younger people. *(This predicts a relationship between increased accidents and aging, as reflexes are slowed or decrease. While this is an inverse relationship, it is indeed a directional relationship.)*

A **nondirectional hypothesis** shows just the opposite; it shows that no direction exists between the variables. For example:

- There is a relationship between diet and the risk of obesity. *(This does not clearly predict a direction, whereas the following statement would.)*
- People who consume more than 3,000 calories per day will have an increased risk of being obese. *(This shows a relationship between increased caloric consumption and increased risk of being obese, and an obvious direction.)*

Fast Facts

The purpose of research questions is to generate new knowledge, whereas the purpose of EBP questions is to make decisions about factors that affect patient care.

Research questions are statements that seek to address an identified research problem. In some cases, they are a direct rewording of the statement of purpose phrased as a question rather than a statement (Polit & Beck, 2016). For example, if the problem statement is to determine the difference between high-carbohydrate diets and obesity, the purpose may be to examine the link between these elements. The research question(s) may be:

- Is there a correlation between diets of complex carbohydrates and increased obesity?
- Is there a decreased incidence of obesity among people who do not consume carbohydrates?
- Is there a family history that predisposes one to obesity?

Answers to the following queries can be used to develop research questions:

- Is there a relationship?
- What is the direction of the relationship?
- What is the strength of the relationship?
- What is the type of the relationship?

Step Nine: Identify the Type of Research Design

The most basic way of identifying the type of research design is to **ask if it is quantitative or qualitative**. Then, look at the factors for each type of study that will need to be addressed, including the population, how the data will be analyzed, and the communication of the results. These topics are discussed in greater detail in Chapter 8, Evaluating the Evidence, and Chapter 9, Barriers to Disseminating the Evidence.

Fast Facts

Florence Nightingale, although not an evidence-based researcher, is credited as the first nurse researcher because of her observations and notes made during the Crimean War. The two basic types of research are quantitative and qualitative. Each category includes multiple types of research. The basic steps in the research process are as follows: (1) identify the problem to be examined (problem statement); (2) state the purpose of the study; (3) determine the study variables; (4) conduct a review of the literature; (5) identify a theoretical or conceptual framework; (6) conduct the study ethically; (7) identify study assumptions; (8) formulate the hypothesis or research questions (what it is the researcher wants to know or predict); and (9) identify the type of research design you want to use. Although these steps are not the only way to conduct research, they provide a framework to guide you as you begin to understand the research process.

REFERENCES

Adams, S. (2009). Identifying research questions. In N. A. Schmidt & J. M. Brown (Eds.), *Evidence-based practice for nurses: Appraisal and application of research* (pp. 57–74). Boston, MA: Jones & Bartlett.

Barone, S., Roy, C., & Frederickson, K. (2008). Instruments used in Roy adaptation model-based research: Review, critique and further directions. *Nursing Science Quarterly, 21*(4), 353–362. doi:10.1177/0894318408323491

Fain, J. A. (2009). *Reading, understanding, and applying nursing research* (3rd ed.). Philadelphia, PA: F. A. Davis.

Fawcett, J. (1999). *The relationship between theory and research*. Philadelphia, PA: F. A. Davis.

Gillis, A., & Jackson, W. (2002). *Research for nurses: Methods and interpretation*. Philadelphia, PA: F. A. Davis.

Houser, J. (2008). *Nursing research: Reading, using, and creating evidence.* Sudbury, MA: Jones & Bartlett.

Kolcaba, K. (2019). The comfort line. Retrieved from https://www.thecom fortline.com/

LoBiondo-Wood, G., & Haber, J. (2014). *Nursing research: Methods and critical appraisal for evidence based practice* (8th ed.). St. Louis, MO: Mosby.

McEwen, M., & Wills, E. M. (2002). *Theoretical basis for nursing.* Philadelphia, PA: Lippincott, Williams & Wilkins.

Meleis, A. I. (2007). *Theoretical nursing: Development and progress* (4th ed.). Philadelphia, PA: Lippincott, Williams & Wilkins.

Nieswiadomy, R. M. (2012). *Foundations of nursing research* (6th ed.). Upper Saddle River, NJ: Pearson.

Polit, D. F., & Beck, C. T. (2016). *Nursing research: Generating and assessing evidence for nursing practice* (10th ed.). Philadelphia, PA: Wolters Kluwer.

Schmidt, N. A., & Brown, J. M. (Eds.). (2009). *Evidence-based practice for nurses: Appraisal and application of research.* Sudbury, MA: Jones & Bartlett.

5

Quantitative Research

The two main research designs are quantitative and qualitative. This chapter discusses the basics of quantitative research designs. Chapter 6, Qualitative Research, discusses the basics of qualitative research designs. Quantitative research has many designs, and the literature on the subject is vast. This chapter provides a brief overview of basic quantitative research designs, along with related key terminology needed to understand the basics of evidence-based practice (EBP). For further clarification of topics and concepts, consult a comprehensive and detailed nursing research textbook.

In this chapter, you will learn:

1. A basic overview of quantitative research
2. The two basic designs of quantitative research: experimental and nonexperimental
3. The Hawthorne effect
4. Randomization
5. How to complete a basic analysis of findings in quantitative research

QUANTITATIVE RESEARCH

Quantitative research designs examine relationships between variables and are categorized as experimental or nonexperimental. In experimental designs, the researcher usually manipulates the

Table 5.1

Experimental and Nonexperimental Quantitative Research Designs

Experimental Designs	Nonexperimental Designs
■ True experimental design	■ Descriptive studies
■ Pretest–posttest control group	■ Action studies
■ Posttest-only control group	■ Comparative studies
■ Solomon four group	■ Correlational studies
■ Quasi-experimental designs	■ Developmental studies
■ Nonequivalent control group	■ Evaluation studies
■ Factorial	■ Meta-analysis studies
■ Randomized block	■ Methodological studies
■ Crossover/repeated measures	■ Needs-assessment studies
■ Time series	■ Secondary analysis studies
■ Preexperimental	■ Survey studies

experimental variables, there is a comparison group in the study, and the subjects are usually randomly assigned to the experimental or to the comparison group. The nonexperimental design is used when research cannot be conducted on human subjects because it would either be unethical or cause pain or harm to the subjects. Nonexperimental designs are descriptive and describe the phenomenon as it exists. The researcher does not have control over the subjects and can only attempt to control for extraneous variables by carefully selecting the study sample. For a brief overview of experimental and nonexperimental designs, see Table 5.1.

DESIGNS IN QUANTITATIVE RESEARCH

Experimental Designs

True Experimental Design

In a true experimental design, the researcher has greater control over the situation because the rival or alternative hypothesis can be ruled out as an explanation for the observed response (Fain, 2009). Three criteria are necessary for a true experimental design:

1. The researcher manipulates the experimental variables.
2. At least one experimental and one comparison group are included in the study.
3. Subjects are randomly assigned to either the experimental or the comparison group.

The researcher also looks for a cause and effect (outcome). **All experimental studies involve the manipulation of the independent variable (cause) and, then, the measurement of the dependent variable (effect).** Several issues related to experimental design need to be mentioned. The first is that not all variables can be manipulated. For example, if you are studying patients who have pneumonia, the researcher cannot infect more patients with pneumonia so that they can be added to the study. That would not be ethical. So, when conducting an experimental research study or when reading a study to determine to what extent the researcher was able to control the variables involved, keep these points in mind.

Fast Facts

All experimental studies involve the manipulation of the independent variable and, then, the measurement of the dependent variable.

Determining whether a study is ethical is very important. In the past, some studies were conducted without regard to human rights. The famous Tuskegee syphilis study is one such example. This study involved an experiment that lasted more than 40 years. It was designed to examine the long-term effects of syphilis in adult African American men, but many of the men studied were not aware that they were subjects. This violates the right of informed consent. In addition, when penicillin became available to treat syphilis, the government withheld the medication from this group so that the study could continue. Without the penicillin, many of the men died. Since that time, legislation has imposed important safeguards to prevent such an atrocity from happening again (Nieswiadomy, 2012). Today, subjects in every study must give informed consent. This means that before a researcher begins collecting data, he or she must make sure that each participant understands the nature of the research project and the implications of participating in the study. The researcher must provide information about the potential benefits and risks and ensure that the subject is participating voluntarily, without any coercion. Researchers also must also provide ample time for the subjects to ask questions and clarify any confusion about participation in the study. For children, a parent or custodian must give consent for the child to participate.

"First, do no harm," the most basic principle of medicine, applies to research as well as to the practice of medicine. In the research environment, it simply means that no subject shall be harmed during the process of data collection. This is extremely important. Consent to conduct a study must also be obtained from an institution's internal review board, known as an institutional review board (IRB). The IRB is a group of individuals who review and approve all studies before they are conducted. This ensures that human rights are protected and proper procedures or protocols are being followed so that no participant is harmed.

Fast Facts

Subjects in every study must give informed consent.

For a **retrospective study,** researchers **look back in time to data already obtained** and on record. In most cases, regulations requiring informed consent do not apply, as long as the data do not identify the patient. However, the U.S. Health Insurance Portability and Accountability Act (HIPAA) of 1996 is very clear about the type of information that can be removed from patient records for the data to be considered de-identified (Polit & Beck, 2016). HIPAA requires national standards for electronic medical information to keep health information private. An institution, such as a hospital, can disclose individually identifiable health information (IIHI) from its records if a patient signs an authorization allowing access. This authorization can be incorporated within a consent form, or it can be a separate document (Polit & Beck, 2016). It is best to check with each institution as to its policies and procedures before looking at any patient data.

The **Hawthorne effect is an important phenomenon in experimental designs.** It refers to how participants in a study react as a consequence of being studied. If a researcher is conducting a study and the subjects know they are being studied, they may change their behavior, actions, or replies to questions during the study. That change of behavior is the Hawthorne effect. For example, suppose a nurse is conducting a study on the handwashing compliance of staff and is observing members of the staff walking in and out of patient rooms. The staff may become suspicious as to why the researcher is watching them. They may fear the researcher is monitoring their practices and, therefore, change their behavior and wash their hands more frequently than they normally would have done. This skews the results of the study. Waltz, Strickland, and Lenz (2005) note that subjects who are being observed usually notice the observer's presence and figure out they are being watched within approximately 10 minutes.

Fast Facts

The Hawthorne effect occurs when subjects change their behavior, actions, or responses to questions because they know they are being studied.

For a good experimental study to be conducted, there also needs to be randomization. **Randomization** is a procedure that **ensures that every subject has an equal chance of being chosen** for the experiment. There are numerous methods to achieve this goal. It can be done by computer-generated numbers, a random numbers chart, selection of every third person, or a simple flip of a coin. An experimental study usually has two separate groups of subjects: a true experimental group and a control group. When applying a variable, or intervention of interest, such as testing a new drug and its effects, the members of the experimental group would receive the drug, and the members of the control group would not. The control group might also be referred to as the comparison group. To alleviate the Hawthorne effect, the researcher may choose to "blind" the study. **Blinding occurs when subjects do not know whether they are in the experimental group or the control group.** For example, if the researcher is testing a new medication for depression, the subjects will not know if they are getting the new medication or a placebo, which is a nontherapeutic (pretend, or fake) medication. A study can be single blinded or double blinded. Single blinding is a one-way process in which the subject does not know if he or she is in the experimental or control group. Double blinding is a two-way process that exists when neither the researcher nor the subject knows if the subject is in the experimental group or in the control group. In the preceding example, neither the researcher nor the subjects would know who is receiving the medication and who is receiving the placebo. **Double blinding is the most efficient way to eliminate any type of subjectivity or bias.** *Bias* is an important term that **means an influence of some sort on the study or outcome of the study.** This occurs when the researcher interjects his or her personal beliefs into the study, either knowingly or unknowingly. For example, assume a researcher is studying the positive effects of using sugar to sweeten coffee. First, the researcher is guilty of bias in the way the study is worded. It states a "positive" effect. How does the researcher know it will be positive? Second, the researcher may say to the subject, "Doesn't your coffee taste sweeter and better?" In this case, the researcher is planting ideas into the subject's head and altering the outcome of the experiment. That is a form of bias.

Double blinding is the most efficient way to eliminate any type of subjectivity or bias.

Sampling

For evidence-based research, the "P" or population of interest in a PICOT question is the entire group of interest. (See Chapter 2, Asking the Compelling Question, for an explanation of the PICOT method.) Sampling is a critical part of the design. **Sampling** involves selecting a part of the population to represent the population. A **sample** is a subset of the population. Researchers typically work with samples rather than populations for reasons of practicality. In quantitative research a representative sample is one whose characteristics closely match those of the population. **Sampling bias** occurs when a segment of the population is either overrepresented or underrepresented (Polit & Beck, 2016).

Another type of sampling is **convenience sampling**. This entails selecting the most conveniently available people as participants. An example would be a nurse who needs 50 burn patient participants and chooses the first 50 people who are admitted to the hospital with a burn injury. These participants are chosen because they are convenient, in that they are in the hospital with a burn injury. They do not need to be recruited or sought out. The problem with this type of sampling is that the representation of people (participants) may not be indicative of all people in the population. Those who are selected for study are chosen because they are very easy to use, but this approach makes the representative sample very weak.

Purposive sampling is based on the researcher's knowledge about a population. The researcher decides to select people who are believed to be particularly knowledgeable about a specific issue being studied. They are purposely chosen. This can lead to bias (Polit & Beck, 2016).

Probability sampling involves a random selection of people from a population. It is not the same as random assignment frequently used in randomized controlled trials (RCTs). In **random sampling**, each person in the population has an equal, independent chance of being selected. **Random assignment** to different treatment conditions has no bearing on how participants in the RCT were selected (Polit & Beck, 2016). It just describes how they are assigned to a treatment group or a control group.

Nonprobability sampling differs from probability sampling in that samples are rarely representative of the population. If every person in the sampling population does not have an equal chance of being chosen, it is likely that some segment or part of the population will be underrepresented (Polit & Beck, 2016).

Systematic sampling involves choosing every nth case from a list, such as every 10th person on a patient list. So, if you want to select 100 people for a study, you would choose number 10 on a list of patient names and then continue to choose numbers 20, 30, 40, and so on until reaching 100. The **sampling interval** is the interval at which the participants are selected, such as every 5th person, every 10th person, or whatever the researcher decides. So, this is simply the interval or number chosen. In the preceding example, the sampling interval would be 10, for every 10th person.

In choosing participants for a study, researchers often specify inclusion or exclusion criteria. **Inclusion criteria** are what qualify a person to be part of the study. **Exclusion criteria** are what exclude a person from being part of a study. Let's say you want to conduct an EBP project focusing on a population of nurses, including those with a doctoral degree. The project would include nurses with and without doctoral degrees. It would exclude nonnurses and those with a doctoral degree who are not nurses. It is important, when looking at who is included or excluded from a study, to evaluate whether the population or sample is evenly, fairly, and adequately represented or constitutes a nonrepresentative sample.

Quasi-Experimental Design

In a quasi-experimental design, which is similar to an experimental design, **there is no randomization or comparison group**. This type of study might be conducted when randomization is not possible. The researcher uses an already established group for the experimental group. This type of design is used with people in their naturally occurring groups, which is more like the "real world." For example, a researcher studying a group of Native Americans is working with a group that is predetermined by culture. This makes determining the cause-and-effect relationship weaker than in a true experimental design because the researcher is making generalizations about only one group of individuals, Native Americans. The researcher cannot assume that these findings would also be applicable to, say, African Americans. As a result, quasi-experimental designs are ranked lower on the hierarchy of rating evidence for EBP.

Nonexperimental Designs

A nonexperimental design is frequently used when experimental research cannot be conducted on human subjects. For example, suppose a researcher wants to study the effects of pain on children. It would be unethical to induce pain in asymptomatic children to conduct the study. The researcher cannot intentionally subject any one group to pain. All nonexperimental studies are therefore descriptive in nature. Because the researcher cannot manipulate or control variables, he or she can only describe the phenomena as they exist. The researcher can, however, try to control extraneous variables by carefully selecting the study sample. An extraneous variable is one that is not of interest to the researcher but can affect the study by causing an unanticipated effect. These are also called intervening, or confounding, variables. The two broad categories of nonexperimental design are descriptive and correlational. These are discussed below, along with survey studies, comparative studies, and methodological studies.

Descriptive Design Studies

Descriptive design studies describe in detail the phenomenon of interest and the relationship among its variables. The purpose of descriptive designs is to observe and describe phenomena in real-life situations. In nursing, a descriptive design can be used to identify problems, make decisions, or determine what other people in similar situations are doing (Houser, 2008). For a descriptive study, information already exists in the literature about the phenomenon of interest, whereas for an exploratory study, no such information is available. An example of an **exploratory study** would be a researcher studying the use of a particular antibiotic, let's say antibiotic X. If antibiotic X is given intravenously, the researcher's question would be "Does it cause venous irritation?" The researcher would describe what happens, if anything, when the antibiotic is given. The researcher is exploring a new situation and gathering new data and has no knowledge of a possible answer based on published reports. This is an exploratory study.

Remember that if the study is observational or descriptive in nature, the characteristics of the sample group are usually examined by methods such as questionnaires, surveys, interviews, and direct observation. Conclusions are made about the subjects or sample from these observations. The sample is usually divided, but this may not be done randomly (Carlson, Kruse, & Rouse, 1999).

Correlational Design Studies

Correlational design studies are used to find relationships between two or more variables within a situation without knowing the reason for the relationship (Boswell & Cannon, 2007). In correlational studies, the researcher seeks to find the strength of the relationship between variables to see if a change in one variable results in a change in the other, that is, to see if there is a correlation between the two variables. The magnitude or direction of a correlation can be measured by using a positive or negative correlation coefficient. Coefficients range from -1.00 (a negative correlation) to 1.00 (a positive correlation). A correlation coefficient of 0.00 shows no relationship between the variables. Correlation coefficients can be reported through various statistics, such as Pearson's product moment correlation or Spearman's rho (Nieswiadomy, 2012). In reviewing evidence from a correlational study, keep in mind that a correlation does not prove causality. In other words, just because a correlation was found between A and B does not mean that A caused B. Correlational research simply seeks to find the "correlation."

Survey Studies

Survey studies obtain data through subjects' self-reporting about variables such as attitudes, perceptions, and behaviors. Surveys can be conducted face to face or over the telephone. Using questionnaires is a popular method in collecting data (Peters, 2009). Survey tools are readily available, or the researcher may choose to develop his or her own. If the researcher develops a new survey tool, he or she must be sure to test the new tool in a pilot study to confirm that it is valid and reliable. A **pilot study is a small-scale trial run** of a larger research project using a smaller number of subjects. In this case, the pilot study would be done to test the survey tool. Many of us could have received surveys in the mail. **Cross-sectional surveys look at people at one point in time; longitudinal surveys follow subjects over a period of time.**

Some advantages of surveys are that the researcher can collect a large amount of information quickly at a minimal cost. Using survey tools, a researcher can reach large groups of people in a shorter amount of time than is possible when conducting a face-to-face survey. Incentives may be offered for the participant to complete the survey. Short surveys are usually more effective than long and detailed surveys.

Comparative Studies

Comparative studies look at the difference between intact groups on some dependent variable of interest. Although this sounds a lot like a true experimental study, the difference is in the extent to which the researcher can manipulate the independent variable. In comparative studies, there is no manipulation of the independent variable. For example, when looking at spousal abuse, it would not be ethical to examine abuse as an independent variable in one group and then choose another group whose members would not be abused.

Comparative studies frequently are classified as retrospective or prospective. In retrospective studies, the researcher looks backward in time. In prospective studies, the researcher looks for an effect in "real time" or in the future.

Methodological Studies

In methodological studies, nurse researchers are looking at the method. This type of study is used most often to test instruments or analyze the development, testing, and evaluation of research instruments. For example, assume a researcher develops a tool to measure "happiness" in obstetric patients after delivery. The new "happiness scale" would need to be tested to see if it is indeed a valid method of measuring happiness. This would be done in a methodological study. Remember the researcher is just testing the method.

A biophysiological method tests an instrument used for collecting biophysiological data of some kind, such as blood pressure, heart rate, and so on. When obtaining this type of data, it is important that the biophysiological instrument be calibrated to ensure accuracy, reliability, and validity before the study is started. An example of a biophysiological method or an instrument is a glucose meter. If you are conducting a study about glucose levels using a new glucose meter, you would want to ensure that the meter is working properly before conducting the study.

Fast Facts

It is important not to confuse exploratory and explanatory research.

Exploratory research studies are conducted when little is known about the phenomena of interest. For example, a researcher might decide to investigate the needs of the families of patients who are discharged with implanted vagal nerve stimulators. If a review of the literature demonstrates limited information on vagal nerve stimulators, it would be most appropriate to do an exploratory study.

In explanatory research studies, the researcher searches for causal explanations or explanations of "why" or "how" phenomena are related. This method is much more rigorous than exploratory or descriptive research and usually involves experimental-type research. Whereas in exploratory and descriptive studies, the researcher describes phenomena and examines relationships between phenomena, in explanatory research, the researcher provides an explanation for the relationships that are found between phenomena (Nieswiadomy, 2012). For example, in the exploratory research on antibiotic X mentioned earlier, suppose the researcher found that antibiotic X does indeed cause venous irritation. In explanatory research, the researcher explains why the venous irritation happens. In this case, it could be related to the pH of antibiotic X.

ANALYSIS OF FINDINGS IN QUANTITATIVE RESEARCH

The analysis of data, along with both descriptive and inferential statistics, can be overwhelming for a person new to research and goes beyond the scope of this book. More detail on this type of data analysis can be found by consulting a basic research text. A brief explanation of four basic concepts—level of significance, confidence intervals, effect size, and standard deviation—follows. Table 5.2 provides a list of questions to ask in critiquing a quantitative study.

Level of Significance

The level of statistical significance is written in terms of a probability value, commonly abbreviated in research reports as the *p* value. The *p* value measures how much evidence there is against the **null hypothesis** (a finding of no relationship between phenomena), that is, how much of a chance there is that the null hypothesis is wrong. In nursing research, for a result to be considered significant, it must have a *p* value of less than 0.05. **If the *p* value is less than 0.05, the result is significant. If the *p* value is greater than 0.05, the result is not considered significant.**

More simply, if a report indicates that the findings are significant at the 0.05 level, that means that only 5 times out of 100 (5 divided by 100, or 0.05) would the obtained results be incorrect. In other words, 95 out of 100 times, the same results (a positive correlation or relationship) could be obtained with another sample or test. This is the same as saying that a null hypothesis (no correlation or relationship

Table 5.2

Guide to Critiquing Quantitative Research		
Critiquing Guidelines	**YES**	**NO**
Ask yourself:		
What type of quantitative study was done?		
■ Does the process relate to the type of study?	☐	☐
■ Does it make sense?	☐	☐
Was the design of the study identified, and does it fit the hypothesis or answer the research questions?		
■ What design was used?	☐	☐
■ Does it make sense for this type of study?	☐	☐
■ Would this type of study test the hypothesis presented?	☐	☐
What were the results of the study?		
■ How were they obtained and measured statistically?	☐	☐
■ Is this significant?	☐	☐
■ Would the results help locally or impact clinical practice?	☐	☐
Is the measurement reliable?		
■ Does it measure the same thing on repeated measures?	☐	☐
■ Is the study reproducible?	☐	☐
■ Are the results valid?	☐	☐
■ Does the study measure what it was supposed to measure?	☐	☐
■ Is any bias present?	☐	☐
■ Are there any confounding variables?	☐	☐
More Specific Questions	**YES**	**NO**
What is the measurement effect?		
■ How many participants were enrolled in the study? ($n =$ _____)	☐	☐
■ Were the two groups (control and experimental) evenly divided?		
Are the results of the study clinically significant?		
■ If they are significant, at what level of measurement?	☐	☐
How was the sample size decided?		
■ Was there randomization?	☐	☐
■ Was there blinding of the subjects?	☐	☐
How were the data analyzed?		
■ What statistical tests were used, if any?	☐	☐
■ Was there a significant *p* value?	☐	☐

between variables) will be rejected only 5 times. You can have a high degree of confidence that these results are reliable. So a *p* value of less than 0.05 is good. A *p* value of less than 0.01 is better. Look at the *p* values in Table 5.3. Which are less than 0.05?

Keep in mind that while the *p* value tells you that a difference exists between the experimental and control groups, it does not

Table 5.3

Examples of *p* Values and Standard Deviations

Interview No.	Standard Deviation	*p* Value
Interview 1 ($n = 35$)	1.33	.014
Interview 2 ($n = 40$)	1.05	.057
Interview 3 ($n = 50$)	0.91	.008 (significant)
Interview 4 ($n = 34$)	1.00 (good)	.011

tell you the magnitude of the effect. To understand the magnitude of the effect, you would need to understand the clinical and statistical significance, which involves looking at confidence intervals and effect size (Rempher & Silkman, 2007).

Fast Facts

The 95% confidence interval is another commonly used estimate of precision. It is calculated by using the standard deviation to create a range of values that is 95% likely to contain the true population mean.

Confidence Interval

Confidence intervals are computed based on the mean and standard deviation. If a study has a confidence interval (usually abbreviated as CI in research reports) of more than 95%, that is good. This means that the data are correct 95% of the time. So a 99% CI is better than a 90% CI.

Confidence intervals reflect the degree of risk researchers are willing to take of being wrong. With a 95% CI, researchers accept the probability that they will be wrong only 5 times out of 100 (Polit & Beck, 2016).

Effect Size

An effect size is the magnitude of the relationship between two variables, or the magnitude of the difference between two groups with regard to some attribute of interest (Polit & Beck, 2016). Although an intervention or variable is expected to have an impact on the outcome and be reported as clinically significant, this may not translate into actually being clinically significant (Houser, 2008). For example, suppose a researcher is studying the effect of aerobic exercise on heart rate and losing weight. If the relationship is strong, an effect will be seen with a small sample size. However, if it is found that exercise has little effect on the heart rates of patients with hyperthyroidism, a much larger sample will be needed to find any significant changes in heart rate in this study. In other words, when a strong relationship between variables exists, a small sample might be possible to show that relationship. However, when the strength of the relationship between variables is not as strong or when another intervening variable might affect the results, a much larger sample of subjects will be needed.

Standard Deviation

A standard deviation shows the average amount by which values deviate from the mean. The mean is simply the average of a set of numbers. For example, if you add 10, 11, and 12, you come up with 33. If you then divide that sum (33) by the total numbers in the example (3), your mean, or average, is 11. The standard deviation (usually abbreviated as SD in research reports) is a useful variability index for describing a distribution and interpreting individual scores in relation to other scores in the sample. Similar to the mean, the SD is a stable estimate of a parameter and is the preferred way of determining a distribution's variability. This is only appropriate for variables measured on an interval or ratio scale.

When researchers consider an analysis that reports an SD, they are looking for a result as close to the number 1 as possible. It can be positive or negative. So, an SD of +0.9 is good. An SD of +3.0 is worse. An SD of −1.0 is good, but an SD of −5.7 is bad. The absolute measure is zero, so the closer you get to zero, the better. Table 5.3 provides examples of standard deviation.

Levels of Measurement

According to Polit and Beck (2016), there are four main classes or levels of measurements that involve the use of numbers in reporting results: nominal, ordinal, interval, and ratio measurement. **Nominal measurement** is the lowest level and involves using numbers to categorize attributes. For example, a researcher might code males as "1" and females as "2." These numbers have no quantitative meaning.

Ordinal measurement ranks a subject based on a relative standing or attribute. An example would be assigning the following numbers to a person's ability to comb his or her hair: 4 = completely independent, 3 = needs minimal assistance; 2 = needs maximal assistance, 1 = needs complete assistance. Ordinal measurement does not tell us how much greater one level is than another. In the preceding example, we do not know whether or not being completely independent is twice as good as needing maximal assistance.

Interval measurement occurs when researchers can rank subjects based on a particular attribute and can specify the distance between them. Suppose you are being graded on a standard test and the highest grade you can get is 100. While a grade of 100 is higher than 80, the difference between 100 and 80 is the same as that between 80 and 60. When researchers use this type of ranking, the interval measurements can be averaged. There are several statistical procedures that require interval data.

Ratio measurement is the highest level of measurement. Ratio scales differ from interval scales in that they have a meaningful zero. A common example is ambient temperature as measured on a standard thermometer. Both Fahrenheit and Celsius thermometers consist of a scale for measuring temperature (interval measurement). In these scales, zero on the thermometer does not indicate the absence of heat; it is just a set point. Furthermore, it would be inaccurate to say that 40° is twice as hot as 20°.

Fast Facts

The two main types of research are quantitative and qualitative. Quantitative research is further divided into experimental and nonexperimental. A variable is something that can be measured, such as blood pressure or heart rate. The independent variable influences the dependent variable. The independent variable is the "cause," and the dependent variable is the "effect." Randomization is a method used to choose subjects for a study. With randomization, every subject or participant has an equal chance of being selected. Bias occurs when researchers interject their feelings or personal beliefs into the study in a way that might affect the outcome of the study. Retrospective studies look backward in time, and prospective studies look at issues in "real time" or in the future.

REFERENCES

Boswell, C., & Cannon, S. (Eds.). (2007). *Introduction to nursing research: Incorporating evidence-based practice*. Sudbury, MA: Jones & Bartlett.

Carlson, D. S., Kruse, L. K., & Rouse, C. L. (1999). Critiquing nursing research. A user friendly guide for the staff nurse. *Journal of Emergency Nursing, 25*(4), 330–332. doi:10.1016/S0099-1767(99)70064-4

Fain, J. A. (2009). *Reading, understanding, and applying nursing research* (3rd ed.). Philadelphia, PA: F. A. Davis.

Houser, J. (2008). *Nursing research: Reading, using, and creating evidence.* Sudbury, MA: Jones & Bartlett.

Nieswiadomy, R. M. (2012). *Foundations of nursing research* (6th ed.). Upper Saddle River, NJ: Pearson.

Peters, R. M. (2009). Quantitative designs: Using numbers to provide evidence. In N. A. Schmidt & J. M. Brown (Eds.), *Evidence-based practice for nurses: Appraisal and application of research* (pp. 57–74). Boston, MA: Jones & Bartlett.

Polit, D. F., & Beck, C. T. (2016). *Nursing research: Generating and assessing evidence for nursing practice* (10th ed.). Philadelphia, PA: Wolters Kluwer.

Rempher, K. J., & Silkman, C. (2007). How to appraise quantitative research articles. *American Nurse Today, 2*(1), 26–28. Retrieved from https://www.americannursetoday.com/how-to-appraise-quantitative-research-articles

Waltz, C. F., Strickland, O. L., & Lenz, E. R. (2005). *Measurement in nursing research* (3rd ed.). New York, NY: Springer Publishing.

6

Qualitative Research

Of the two main types of research design introduced in earlier chapters, qualitative research is the more subjective. In contrast to quantitative research, which involves datasets of numbers, qualitative research is more likely to be based on life experiences. It involves smaller groups of subjects, often includes narratives, and attempts to identify common themes. The researcher collects data until saturation is achieved. This chapter explores the characteristics of four types of qualitative research designs: phenomenological, ethnological, grounded theory, and historical. Case studies, narratives, feminist research, and community-based participatory action research are other types of qualitative research.

In this chapter, you will learn:

1. The basic principles of qualitative research
2. How to examine the process of knowing
3. How to explore the basic types of qualitative research, which include:
   - Phenomenology
   - Ethnography
   - Grounded theory
   - Historical research
4. How to examine other examples of qualitative studies, including case studies, community-based participatory action research, feminist research, and narrative research

WHAT IS QUALITATIVE RESEARCH?

Qualitative research is not easily defined. It requires an examination of the quality of something rather than its quantifiable elements. It implies a subjective interpretation. LoBiondo-Wood and Haber (2014) note that qualitative research is about human experiences. It frequently is conducted in natural settings and uses words or text rather than numerical data to describe the experiences being studied.

Before the 1970s, qualitative methods were used primarily in anthropology and sociology. Then, during the 1970s and 1980s, qualitative research methods were adopted by researchers in education, social work, management, nursing, and women's studies (Tilley, 2007). **Qualitative research lends itself effectively to the nursing process, which focuses on the person as a whole.** Over the years, its methods have become valued in the science of nursing, as the nursing process looks at the continuum of care from assessment to diagnosis to planning to interventions to an evaluation of care given.

Clearly, not everything a nurse experiences can be reduced to numbers and physiological measurement. The experienced nurse knows that there is more to nursing that is sometimes left unsaid and unexplained.

Fast Facts

Qualitative research requires an examination of the quality of something rather than its quantifiable elements. It lends itself effectively to the nursing process, which focuses on the body, mind, and spirit of the individual.

THE PROCESS OF KNOWING

How does a nurse "know" or sense when a patient is going to "crash" or deteriorate? How does a patient "get the feeling" that he or she is going to die? Sometimes, nurses just know, but how does one get to this place of knowing? Is it through learning or acquiring facts? Is it instinctive? Or is it something more? Most important, how can it be measured in the research process?

Have you ever cared for a patient and just "sensed" that something was wrong? How did you know? Was it a feeling—a sometimes overwhelming feeling? Perhaps you have worked in the ED or in the ICU. If so, have you experienced the feeling that your patient was going to crash or was about to die? How and why did you get that feeling? How did you know? How can you measure that?

Michael Polanyi: Tacit Knowledge

Michael Polanyi, a professor of physical chemistry and social science, made significant contributions to the fields of philosophy and social science. He referred to this type of personal knowing as *tacit knowledge*. He believed that creative acts (especially acts of discovery) are shot through, or charged, with strong personal feelings and commitments (personal knowledge). Polanyi said that these personal hunches, informed guesses, and imaginings are part of exploratory acts that are motivated by what he called passions. He felt these "hunches," which form a prelogical phase, occurred because we "knew more than we could tell" (Smith, 2003). It is an interesting concept to explore. More information about Polanyi's ideas can be found on the web at polanyisociety.org.

Barbara Carper: Patterns of Knowing

To explain how we know what we know, Barbara Carper (1978) examined four types, or patterns, of knowing: empirical, personal, ethical, and aesthetic. Empirical knowledge is what we know through our physical senses. This is something we can hear, touch, taste, and see. Investigations of these areas are best handled through quantitative methods of discovery. Personal knowledge concerns the inner experience we have. It is the shared human experience and humanistic qualities of knowing. Ethical knowledge requires that we make moment-to-moment decisions about what is right, what should be done, and what is good. This knowledge directs our personal conduct. Aesthetic knowledge is abstract and gives us an appreciation of the deeper meaning of the situation. It takes an inductive approach to knowledge acquisition. These four patterns of knowing make it evident that the nurse who wants to research aesthetic knowing, in particular, will find a qualitative method more appropriate than a quantitative method.

Fast Facts

Barbara Carper's four types of knowledge are empirical, personal, ethical, and aesthetic.

TYPES OF QUALITATIVE RESEARCH

Although many types of qualitative research can be conducted, only the four main types are discussed here. In qualitative research, the people who are being studied are called "participants" or "informants" rather than "subjects," which is the term more frequently used in quantitative research.

When planning a qualitative study, it is important to consider exactly what you are interested in studying or exploring. Table 6.1 presents a decision path that can provide guidance in choosing the correct type of qualitative research to use. Keep in mind that for an evidence-based project, you will not conduct an actual research study but rather gather "evidence" to examine your topic of interest.

Qualitative research does not begin with a hypothesis. The researcher does not begin such a study by predicting the results. In a qualitative study, the researcher in effect becomes the research tool

Table 6.1

Qualitative Research Decision Path		
If You Are Interested in:	**Method to Consider Is:**	**A Question to Ask Might Be:**
Understanding the personal and human experience ⟹	Phenomenology ⟹	What is the "lived experience"?
Uncovering a social experience ⟹	Grounded theory ⟹	How does this social group react to…?
Learning about how a culture responds, feels, and reacts ⟹	Ethnography ⟹	How does this cultural group view or perceive caring?
Understanding the past through collection, organization, and critical appraisal of the facts ⟹	Historical research ⟹	What caused an outbreak of polio in the past that may contribute to the outbreaks of today?
Obtaining unique stories and examples ⟹	Case study ⟹	How do Native Americans value healthcare?
Exploring the gender domination and discrimination within patriarchal societies ⟹	Feminist research ⟹	How do women make decisions?

or instrument. To avoid bias, the researcher should be free of precon- ceived notions (this can be achieved by bracketing, described later) and be "decentered" so he or she can become immersed in the situation. To accomplish this, a researcher must clear his or her mind and put per- sonal thinking aside. Otherwise, bias may become part of the study.

One way that a qualitative researcher gathers information is through interviews. While conducting an interview, the researcher may collect field notes by using a recording device or taking notes to ensure accurate recall of statements, thoughts, and information gathered. An interview may contain too much information for the researcher to trust to memory. These notes may be written during the interview session, if not too distracting for the participant, or may be written after the interview is completed. Sometimes during the interview, unusual mannerisms are present. It may be important for the researcher to include these mannerisms in his or her field notes. For example, if during an entire interview, the informant is wringing his or her hands and sweating profusely, the researcher should record this in a field note since this might signify nervousness or tenseness.

Fast Facts

- In a qualitative study, the researcher becomes the research tool or instrument.
- A researcher must clear his or her mind and put personal thinking aside.
- Field notes about an interview help the researcher remember the essential facts.

Phenomenology

Phenomenology is a method that explores the meaning of human experience through the lived experience of the individual. The researcher seeks to use dialogue to explore the meaning that experi- ences hold for each participant. It examines the "humanness" in life. It is important to note that the participants or informants are asked to describe their experiences as *they* perceive them. The researcher must separate out his or her own feelings and not impose them on the research participants—a process known as **bracketing**. This involves the researcher identifying his or her preconceived beliefs and opin- ions about the phenomenon being studied. In phenomenology, the main data are collected during in-depth conversations, which researchers use to try to understand the participant's experience of his or her world (Polit & Beck, 2016). A research question based on phenomenology might be worded something like this: "What is the lived experience of women in abusive relationships?"

Writing the Open-Ended Question

In a phenomenological study, the research question guides the entire study, so it must be worded correctly, focused, and open ended. The question asks about human experiences in a given situation. This question is not exactly the same as the first question or any question used to initiate the dialogue with the participant. For example, although the research question may be "What is the lived experience of women in abusive relationships?" the statement or question that will initiate the dialogue with the participant could be "Tell me what it is like to live with your husband" or "What is your relationship like?" It is important to avoid imposing bias into an opening question. Therefore, an inappropriate question would be "Could you tell me what it is like to live in an abusive relationship?" This particular question assumes and makes a judgment that the relationship is abusive. Although the relationship may be abusive, it is not the researcher's place to tell or suggest to the participant that the relationship is abusive.

Purposive Sampling

Where does one select the sample for a phenomenological study? The researcher will need to engage in purposive sampling. In this type of sampling, the researcher uses his or her own judgment in selecting people who will be representative of the group the researcher is interested in exploring. For example, a researcher might go to a battered woman's shelter to study the lived experiences of women in abusive relationships. The researcher would not go to a church recreation social or a marriage encounter weekend getaway, where the chance of finding participants who are abused might be low. Rather, he or she would go to a place where the population of interest would likely be found.

Sometimes the researcher needs a key informant to begin this process. **A key informant is a person who is knowledgeable about**

the population of interest. This type of research aide is also used in ethnographic studies. The informant might also be able to provide the researcher with access to the designated population. In the preceding example, the key informant might be the director of the woman's shelter, who has known the women for quite some time. If the director introduces the researcher to the women, the women may open up more readily to the researcher.

The researcher should spend time at the place of interest, in this case a woman's shelter, so that the participants or informants get to know and learn to trust the researcher. This process is called **immersion.** The researcher must become immersed in the population of interest to fully gain insight and understanding into what it is like to experience the lived experience being studied. It is hard to understand anything that is being said if, for example, you do not know the language. So, it is important for the researcher to become fully immersed in the population of interest to understand that population.

Fast Facts

To select an appropriate sample:

- Go to a place where the population of interest will likely be found.
- Find a key informant, a person who is knowledgeable about the population of interest.
- Immerse yourself in the population of interest.

Mode of Data Collection

Data may be collected in a number of ways. **In-depth interviews are usually the primary way in which phenomenological data are obtained.** These interviews may be audiotaped or videotaped depending on the informants' comfort level. The data acquired must then be transcribed. Because this work is tedious, it is often done by a hired transcriptionist rather than by the researcher. Once the data have been transcribed, similar or common themes are identified. The researcher can accomplish this through the use of note cards or notes or a computer program designed to make this part of data collection and analysis easier. Commonly used programs include NVivo, NUDIST, and ATLAS.ti.

The researcher continues to collect data until a point of saturation is reached. **Saturation** occurs when common themes are found and no new information is obtained. In the earlier example, suppose the researcher exploring abused women has interviewed six informants, all of whom tell the researcher the same thing: that their significant others often drink alcohol before abusing them. Based on these responses, it may be safe for the researcher to conclude that drinking was a common theme in precipitating abuse of the women. Once saturation of data has occurred, the researcher can stop the interview process. This methodology helps to explain why fewer informants may be needed in a qualitative study. The researcher keeps interviewing informants until saturation is obtained. Saturation could occur after 5 interviews or after 12 or more interviews. In most phenomenological studies, however, the number of participants is usually low.

Ethnography

Ethnography, ethnographic studies, or ethnonursing studies are qualitative studies that explore the cultural aspects of a particular group of informants. Culture refers to the particular way a group of people lives. It is a pattern of human activity reflecting their values and norms. These studies usually require extensive fieldwork (Polit & Beck, 2016). In the United States, ethnography emerged in the early 20th century in the field of cultural anthropology. Margaret Mead is one of the well-known proponents of this type of work (Germain, 2001). **Ethnography seeks to understand the values, norms, customs, rules, and ways of life that categorize the group of interest.** This understanding may take place through conducting interviews, making observations, reading documents, examining photographs, watching videotapes, looking at genograms, or a combination of these approaches. **A genogram is a pictorial diagram of a person's family relationships and medical history.**

Before starting an ethnographic study, bracketing is essential to free yourself of predetermined prejudices or biases. In ethnographic research, immersion is both vital and necessary. The best way for the researcher to understand the culture is to live in the culture. Again, the use of a key informant who assists the researcher in gaining access to the particular group of interest is helpful. It is important to note that a culture does not have to represent a nationality. **A culture can be any group of individuals with similar beliefs, behaviors, rituals, or patterns of life.** For example, a group of mothers who are primary caretakers of children with chronic illnesses can be considered a culture. Nurses can be considered a culture. Also, a culture can contain subcultures. For example, within the culture of the medical profession, nurses, physicians, and nursing assistants or aides can each be considered a subculture. Culture does not necessarily align with one's race (e.g., Caucasian or African American) or place of origin (e.g., Canadian, Lebanese). It can be, but is not necessarily limited to that component.

Ethnographic researchers explore phenomena within a culture from the "**emic**" perspective—an **intrinsic or internal perspective**. For example, a researcher exploring the emic perspective of Native Americans is doing so from the perspective of the Native American. This means that the resulting study would reflect the point of view of Native Americans in giving reasons for their beliefs and customs.

If the researcher were exploring phenomena from an "**etic**" perspective, he or she would be examining the life of the Native American from an **extrinsic or external perspective**. This means that the resulting study would represent the researcher's interpretation of the same Native American customs or beliefs. The etic perspective usually takes on a more analytical perspective.

In ethnographic studies, it is important to do fieldwork or live with the informants in their natural environment. This environment could be people's homes, tribal areas, reservations, huts, or any areas the informant considers home or a place of existing.

Madeleine Leininger has done extensive work in the area of ethnonursing. Her culture care theory was developed in the 1950s and 1960s, and it is expressed visually in the sunrise model. Her 1991 book, *Culture Care Diversity and Universality*, offered a breakthrough concept in exploring the nursing care given to individuals who were culturally different from the nurse caregiver. Her work continued with the development of the theory of transcultural nursing, the purpose of which, Leininger (2002) states, was to discover and explain culturally based factors that influence the health, well-being, illness, or death of individuals of a cultural group. Leininger (1978) also proposed a new method known as *ethnonursing* for nurse researchers to use that includes "the study and analysis of the local or indigenous people's viewpoints, beliefs, and practices about nursing care phenomena and processes of designated cultures" (p. 15). Leininger defines ethnography as "the systematic process of observing, describing, documenting, and analyzing the life ways or particular patterns of culture (or subculture) to grasp the life ways or patterns of the people in their familiar environment" (p. 35). Ethnography and ethnonursing remain valued areas of interest for many nurse researchers.

Fast Facts

Madeleine Leininger applied ethnographic research methods to nursing. She proposed the term *ethnonursing* to describe the study of the nursing practices and beliefs among indigenous people.

Grounded Theory

Grounded theory is a qualitative approach developed by two sociologists: Glaser and Strauss (1967). Using this approach, the researcher studies, collects, and analyzes data before developing a theory grounded in that data (Richards & Morse, 2007). Researchers use grounded theory when they are interested in describing social processes from the perspectives of human interactions or "patterns of action and interaction between and among various types of social units" (Denzin & Lincoln, 1998, p. xx). The goal of grounded theory research is to understand how a group of people defines their reality through social interactions. It uses an inductive (i.e., from the ground up) approach, which relies on everyday behaviors or organizational patterns to generate a theoretical explanation (Munhall, 2001). In this type of study, the researcher uses purposive sampling to look for informants who can shed light on the topic being explored. The emergent theory is based on observations and perceptions of the social scene and evolves during data collection and analysis as a product of the actual research process (Strauss & Corbin, 1994). Data collection is continued until saturation has occurred.

Fast Facts

Grounded theory is an inductive approach to research that uses purposive sampling to find informants who can shed light on the topic of interest.

Historical Research Method

The historical research method is a based on documentation of sources that retrospectively examine events or people (Schmidt & Brown, 2009). This method gains understanding of the past through the collection, organization, and critical appraisal of the facts. One of the main goals of this type of research is to shed light or give a new interpretation on past events. When critiquing this type of study, be aware that the research question may be implied rather than clearly stated. A second important point about historical research is that the more clearly the researcher identifies the historical event being studied, the easier it will be to identify more specific data sources.

In examining the sources of data, it is important to determine whether the data come from primary or secondary sources. **Primary data sources** include eyewitness accounts of the time being studied from those who were actually present (LoBiondo-Wood & Haber, 2014).

Other examples of primary sources include oral histories, written records, diaries, government documents, pictures, relics, artifacts, and physical evidence related to the time specified. **Secondary sources** are second-hand or third-hand accounts of historical events or experiences. They are discussions of events written by individuals who did not actually participate in them but are interpreting or summarizing primary source materials (Polit & Beck, 2016). An example would be an account of an event using an individual's letters (primary sources) as the basis for the interpretation.

Healthcare researchers who conduct historical research in the United States must be aware that the provisions of the Health Insurance Portability and Accountability Act (HIPAA) of 1996 relating to disclosure of medical information and protection of patient privacy have implications for archival as well as present-day studies. HIPAA has raised new barriers for nurse historians seeking to examine archival resources. Access restrictions vary, and nurse historians may not be able to use photographs or images of previous patients that could be construed as violating patient privacy. Researchers must gain permission to access patient records from the 18th century the same way they do for contemporary records. In such cases, however, a waiver of authorization may often be obtained from the institutional review board (IRB; Polit & Beck, 2016).

Fast Facts

The historical research method uses data from primary sources (contemporary records and accounts) or secondary sources (subsequent interpretations of events based on primary sources).

OTHER TYPES OF QUALITATIVE STUDIES

Case Studies

Case studies are in-depth examinations of a single entity or a small group of entities. The entity could be a single person, a family, an institution, a community, or another social unit (Polit & Beck, 2016). A case study examining institutions, for example, might look at facilities such as inpatient psychiatric units. In a case study, the entity is placed center stage for examination. When the case study involves a person, the researcher's focus is to understand why an individual thinks, behaves, or develops in a particular way, often by comparison with his or her status or actions. This type of study usually takes a long time to complete (Polit & Beck, 2016). Researchers using case studies may need to perform multiple in-depth interviews and obtain data from medical records. An example would be an in-depth case study looking at decision making by the parents of an anencephalic infant, who face several tough decisions, including whether to agree to organ donation or to remove the infant born without a brainstem from a ventilator.

There are two types of case studies: intrinsic and instrumental. An **intrinsic case study is used to develop a better understanding of the case**—nothing more or less. The researcher sorts out other curiosities so that the stories of "those living the case" are teased out (Stake, 2000). An example would be the researcher who is studying incarcerated mothers. In an intrinsic case study, the researcher might interview two women who previously participated in a study about drug usage and were now in jail. The researcher would ask them about their lives after being arrested and jailed, seeking insight into the women's experiences. If both women expressed regrets about using drugs and being incarcerated, it could be concluded that these data could guide practice and future research about this issue.

An **instrumental case study selects one case study to illustrate an issue of concern** (Cresswell, 2007). For example, a researcher who would like to challenge the notion that all patients diagnosed with Down syndrome are mentally challenged and of lower intelligence than the general population might focus on one person whose accomplishments belie that notion. In this type of study, the researcher might look at a case in which a person with Down syndrome was not only holding a job but working as the manager at a local restaurant chain. With this evidence in an instrumental case study, the data obtained could be used to change not only perceptions but prejudices and to guide further research.

Community-Based Participatory Action Research

Community-based participatory action research requires that the community actively participate in all stages of the research process (LoBiondo-Wood & Haber, 2014). After identifying a problem, the researcher, together with the community, explores possible solutions, the method of studying the problem, and the analysis of the data obtained. This is an excellent method for solving community-based problems. It proposes that if the community is involved in the process, members may be more apt to "own the project," participate in the project, implement the project, and bring the project to completion or an outcome. An example is research on increased violence in a community related to gangs and drugs. The community comes together with the researcher to determine a plan to address the situation, implement the plan, evaluate the plan, and, in the process, solve or eliminate the problem. If the problem has not been solved or eliminated, perhaps information will have been uncovered that can be used to further assess and develop new solutions.

Feminist Research

This type of research approach focuses on gender domination and discrimination within patriarchal societies. The researcher seeks to establish a nonexploitative relationship with his or her informants and to conduct research that transforms these perceived boundaries (Polit & Beck, 2016). An example of feminist research would be decision making engaged in by postpartum women when choosing whether to breastfeed their babies. Is discrimination involved in their decision-making process? Feminist research seeks to uncover and define these real or perceived boundaries of gender.

Narrative Research or Storytelling

One type of research approach that is gaining in popularity is narratives, or storytelling. This type of research allows people to "tell their stories" so that their motivations, desires, and feelings in a multitude of settings are uncovered. As noted by Polit and Beck (2016), narrative analysis focuses on the story as the object of inquiry to see how individuals make sense of their lives or environment and communicate that meaning through the making of narratives or telling stories.

This method can be very effective with children. For example, Godshall (2013) examined pediatric burn patients who were 5 to 10 years of age and had them color a picture of themselves since their burn injury. The children were then asked to "tell the story" of their picture. This method used the picture as a vehicle to encourage the children to talk not only about their burn injury, but also about what they were thinking and feeling and whether they had learned anything from an age-appropriate teaching/coloring book. It can be difficult to interview children and get them to talk, but if they are asked to color and tell a story, they are often more receptive and able to articulate what they otherwise might not have been able to express.

USES OF QUALITATIVE RESEARCH

Qualitative approaches to research inquiry are a viable way to explore or examine situations or problems that are not easily measured by quantifiable methods. This type of research is growing in popularity and offers nurse researchers a method to use in trying to explain more humanistic situations in which the lived experience of individuals may be influenced by variables not identified through quantitative research. The qualitative approaches mentioned in this chapter, along with others, give nurse researchers the ability to study aspects of life and nursing care requiring abstract thought or in-depth examination of how an individual relates to or fits into the overall healthcare picture. For questions to ask in critiquing a qualitative study, see Table 6.2.

Table 6.2

Guide to Critiquing Qualitative Research

Critiquing Guidelines	YES	NO
Ask yourself:		
What were the results of the study?		
■ Is the phenomenon or topic of interest clearly identified?	☐	☐
■ Does the research approach fit with the purpose or aim of the study?	☐	☐
■ Are the conclusions of the study consistent with the results as reported in the study? (No jumps or reaches for conclusions.)	☐	☐
Are the results valid?		
■ Were the study participants chosen appropriately?	☐	☐
■ Is that consistent with the type of study conducted?	☐	☐
■ Were accuracy and completeness of the study guaranteed?	☐	☐
■ Do the findings fit the data from which they were generated?	☐	☐
Will the results help me take better care of my patients?		
■ Are the findings relevant to people in similar situations?	☐	☐
■ Did the reader learn any new important information?	☐	☐
■ Does the research relate to or change practice?	☐	☐

More Specific Questions	YES	NO
Did the researcher indicate the type of study approach?		
■ Are the language and concepts consistent with the study approach?	☐	☐
■ Are the data collection and data analysis consistent with the study approach?	☐	☐
Is the significance/importance of the study clear?		
■ Does the review of the literature support the need for a study?	☐	☐
■ Does the study make a difference to current practice?	☐	☐

(continued)

Table 6.2

Guide to Critiquing Qualitative Research (*continued*)

More Specific Questions	YES	NO
■ Are the background and significance of the study defined?	☐	☐
■ Are the implications for future research specified?	☐	☐
Is the sampling method clear and appropriate for the type of study?		
■ Does the researcher indicate the sample size and demographics?	☐	☐
■ Does the researcher control the selection of the sample?	☐	☐
■ Is the type of sample appropriate for the type of study?	☐	☐
■ Is the number of sample participants appropriate for the type of study?	☐	☐
Is the way the data were collected clear?		
■ Are the sources and methods of verifying data clear?	☐	☐
■ Are the researcher's roles and actual involvement clearly explained?	☐	☐

Source: Adapted from Melnyk, B. M., & Fineout-Overholt, E. (2010). *Evidence-based practice in nursing & healthcare: A guide to best practice* (2nd ed.). Philadelphia, PA: Lippincott Williams & Wilkins.

Fast Facts

The four patterns of knowing articulated by Carper are empirical knowledge, personal knowledge, ethical knowledge, and aesthetic knowledge. The four main types of qualitative research are phenomenology, ethnography, grounded theory, and historical research. Case studies, narratives or storytelling, feminist research, and community-based participatory action research are other types. The people in a qualitative study are called participants, whereas those in a quantitative study are called subjects. Saturation occurs when all participants in a study are giving the same responses; this is the point at which no new data will be forthcoming. Madeleine Leininger (1991) developed the sunrise model using transcultural nursing, which seeks to discover and explain culturally based factors that influence health, well-being, illness, or death of individuals of a cultural group. Sources of data may be primary or secondary. Primary sources include eyewitness accounts of the event being examined, whereas secondary sources are written by people who heard or read about the event or occurrence from a primary source. Primary sources are much more desirable as accurate accounts of basic information.

REFERENCES

Carper, B. (1978). Fundamental patterns of knowing in nursing. *Advances in Nursing Science, 1*(1), 13–23. Retrieved from https://journals.lww.com/advancesinnursingscience/Citation/1978/10000/Fundamental_Patterns_of_Knowing_in_Nursing.4.aspx

Cresswell, J. W. (2007). *Qualitative inquiry and research design: Choosing among five approaches.* Thousand Oaks, CA: Sage.

Denzin, N. K., & Lincoln, Y. S. (1998). The art and politics of interpretation. In N. K. Denzin & Y. S. Lincoln (Eds.), *Handbook of qualitative research* (2nd ed., pp. 189–192). Thousand Oaks, CA: Sage.

Germain, C. P. (2001). Ethnography. In P. L. Munhall (Ed.), *Nursing research: A qualitative perspective* (pp. 277–306). Boston, MA: Jones & Bartlett.

Glaser, B. G., & Strauss, A. C. (1967). *The discovery of grounded theory: Strategies for qualitative research.* New York, NY: Aldine.

Godshall, M. (2013). *Exploring learning of pediatric burn patients through storytelling.* Unpublished doctoral dissertation, Duquesne University, Pittsburgh, PA.

Leininger, M. (1978). Caring: The essence and central focus of nursing. *The phenomenon of caring.* American Nurses Foundation Nursing Research Report, Part V, 1977.

Leininger, M. (1991). *Culture care diversity and universality.* Sudbury, MA: Jones & Bartlett.

Leininger, M. (2002). Culture care theory: A major contribution to advance transcultural nursing knowledge and practice. *Journal of Transcultural Nursing, 13*(3), 189–192. doi:10.1177/10459602013003005

LoBiondo-Wood, G., & Haber, J. (2014). *Nursing research: Methods and critical appraisal for evidence based practice* (8th ed.). St. Louis, MO: Mosby.

Melnyk, B. M., & Fineout-Overholt, E. (2010). *Evidence-based practice in nursing & healthcare: A guide to best practice* (2nd ed.). Philadelphia, PA: Lippincott Williams & Wilkins.

Munhall, P. L. (2001). *Nursing research: A qualitative perspective* (3rd ed.). Sudbury, MA: Jones & Bartlett.

Polit, D. F., & Beck, C. T. (2016). *Nursing research: Generating and assessing evidence for nursing practice* (10th ed.). Philadelphia, PA: Wolters Kluwer.

Richards, L., & Morse, J. M. (2007). *User's guide to qualitative methods.* Thousand Oaks, CA: Sage.

Schmidt, N. A., & Brown, J. M. (Eds.). (2009). *Evidence-based practice for nurses: Appraisal and application of research.* Sudbury, MA: Jones & Bartlett.

Smith, M. K. (2003). Michael Polanyi and tacit knowledge. Retrieved from http://infed.org/mobi/michael-polanyi-and-tacit-knowledge/

Stake, R. (2000). Case studies. In N. Denzin & Y. Lincoln (Eds.), *Handbook of qualitative research* (2nd ed., pp. 435–454). Thousand Oaks, CA: Sage.

Strauss, A., & Corbin, J. (1994). Grounded theory methodology. In N. K. Denzin & Y. S. Lincoln (Eds.), *Handbook of qualitative research* (pp. 273–285). Thousand Oaks, CA: Sage.

Tilley, D. S. (2007) Qualitative research methods. In C. Boswell & S. Cannon (Eds.), *Introduction to nursing research: Incorporating evidence-based practice* (pp. 193–216). Sudbury, MA: Jones & Bartlett.

7

Finding the Evidence

The two basic formats for articles used for your research evidence are print and electronic. Print sources remain available at most libraries, but most information is now available electronically and is therefore readily accessible to anyone with access to the Internet.

In this chapter, you will learn:

1. The differences between primary, secondary, and tertiary sources
2. How to explore print and electronic sources
3. The basic databases and search engines available when searching for evidence
4. How to conduct a basic literature search

PRIMARY, SECONDARY, AND TERTIARY SOURCES

Primary and secondary data sources were introduced in Chapter 6, Qualitative Research, in the context of qualitative research studies. In conducting research in any field, a primary source is one created by the person or people who conducted the research study or wrote about the topic of interest. It is the original source of the information. Secondary sources are a description of a study or article written by someone else. A secondary source uses information or data from a primary source by describing, summarizing, analyzing, or interpreting the primary source information. For example, a textbook written about nursing education is a primary source. If a person writes a textbook about nursing education and summarizes or describes the information provided in the original textbook, this second textbook is a secondary source. There are also tertiary sources. If the textbook includes other secondary sources explaining nursing education, it then becomes a tertiary source. When searching for evidence, it is preferable to use only primary sources.

PRINT SOURCES

How does one begin to research an evidence-based practice (EBP) project? The **print sources can be found in the library using indexes,** which contain references to articles in periodicals that have been published over a period of years. These print indexes can be used to locate journal articles related to the topic of interest.

Cumulative Index to Nursing and Allied Health Literature

The *Cumulative Index to Nursing and Allied Health Literature* (CINAHL) has been published continuously since 1961. Until 1977, the title was the *Cumulative Index to Nursing Literature*. CINAHL now includes nursing and allied health journals, including dental hygiene, nutrition, occupational therapy, physical therapy, physician's assistant, and respiratory therapy journals. This print index is a bound text found in the periodical section of the library. Do not hesitate to ask the librarian for assistance. Most libraries have research assistants available to help novice researchers. CINAHL is also available online in an electronic database that now is owned and operated by EBSCO Publishing. Information about CINAHL is available at health.ebsco.com/products/the-cinahl-database. A subscription to this database is required, so it is easiest to access through an educational institution or workplace that maintains a subscription. Sometimes, you are able to access full-text articles. In other cases, you will only be able to obtain a reference and an abstract of the article. This varies depending on the type of subscription purchased. Most often references and abstracts are free to the general public without a subscription.

Nursing Studies Index

The *Nursing Studies Index* (NSI) was compiled at the Yale University School of Nursing under the direction of Virginia Henderson. This index is an annotated guide to English-language reports of studies and historical and bibliographical materials about nursing. The four available volumes, published from 1963 to 1972, cover the years 1900 to 1959. This is an important resource for studies conducted during the first 60 years of the 20th century.

National Guideline Clearinghouse: Agency for Healthcare Research and Quality

The Agency for Healthcare Research and Quality (AHRQ) is a free resource providing latest clinical practice guidelines based on scientific evidence. It also contains evidence-based practice center (EBPC) reports. These centers review all relevant scientific literature on a wide spectrum of clinical and health services topics to produce various types of evidence reports. These reports may be used for informing and developing coverage decisions, quality measures, educational materials and tools, clinical practice guidelines, and research agendas. They are available at www.ahrq.gov/research/findings/evidence-based-reports/index.html.

Abstracts

An abstract is a brief summary of an article's content that describes its purpose, methods, major findings, and conclusions. By reading an abstract, the researcher should be able to understand the highlights of the article and determine if it is related to the topic of interest. The abstract, which is usually the first paragraph beneath the title, is identifiable by its appearance; it is usually indented or printed in boldface or italic type. The abstract may be written as one summary paragraph but usually includes subheadings that highlight the research problem or issue addressed, the type of research method used, the results or findings of the study, and the main conclusions or recommendations from the study.

This style of abstract is the basic one you will find provided for a research article. Other styles of abstracts that you may encounter during your search include psychological abstracts, dissertation abstracts, and master's thesis abstracts.

Fast Facts

A database is a collection of data or information stored in a computer system. Think of it as an electronic filing system.

ELECTRONIC SOURCES

Electronic source searches have become the preferred method of accessing research articles and literature. The use of electronic communication has changed the way data are searched for and obtained. Most people today access the world of electronic databases through home computers or personal electronic devices. Schools, universities, and medical institutions also provide access to electronic databases.

Databases

The key to finding data or articles pertinent to your study is to access the appropriate database. There are many to choose from. Some are free, and some must be purchased by universities or medical institutions. For example, MEDLINE can be accessed for free through the National Library of Medicine's PubMed search system. A full bibliographical source is given. Many of the articles thus retrieved are free, but some publishers may charge a fee to purchase a full-text article. See Table 7.1 for examples and descriptions of some common searchable databases.

Bibliographical Sources

A bibliographical source, whether printed or on the web, simply provides you with a complete reference that you can use to locate the full-text article.

Abstracts

As previously noted, an abstract is simply a concise summary of a research article that is designed to help the reader quickly grasp the key elements of the article. Some databases on the web provide free abstracts. Others require you to purchase that information. See Table 7.1 for more information.

Other full-text databases in which you may be interested are:

- **Allied and Complementary Medicine Database (AMED):** The AMED is a bibliographical database produced by the Health Care Information Service of the British Library. It includes journals about complementary medicine and palliative care and can be accessed through EBSCO (see Table 7.1).
- **ClinicalTrials.gov:** This site is provided by the National Institutes of Health (NIH). It is a registry and results database of publicly and privately supported clinical studies conducted around the world. It can be found at www.clinicaltrials.gov.

Table 7.1

Examples of Databases

Database	Description
CINAHL (Cumulative Index of Nursing and Allied Health Literature; 1982–present) ■ Material from more than 3,000 journals ■ Full text is available for more than 300 journals, but it must be purchased ■ Abstracts and bibliographical references are also available ■ Owned and operated by EBSCO Publishing ■ More information is available at health.ebsco.com/products/cinahl-plus-with-full-text	Premier site for nursing and allied health; also includes nutrition, physical therapy, occupational therapy, dentistry, and respiratory therapy journals
DynaMed Plus ■ Evidence-based content/EBSCO ■ Next-generation clinical reference tool	Is a clinical reference tool that clinicians go to for answers; content is written by a world-class team of physicians who synthesize the evidence and provide objective analysis Contains drug information from Micromedex, Canadian, and international guidelines
EBSCOhost is an international information system that provides e-journal, e-book, and print subscriptions as well as e-resource and management tools, full-text and secondary databases, and related services ■ More than 300 full-text or secondary databases are available ■ Includes bibliographical citations, abstracts, and full-text articles and provides other references where the article is cited ■ Multilanguage health databases are available ■ Free trials are available, but they must be purchased ■ More information and a downloadable brochure are available at https://connect.ebsco.com/s/article/EBSCO-eBooks-Promotion-Kit?language=en_US	Provides clinical patient-oriented, administrative databases with the latest bedside evidence, nursing resources, education materials, marketing tools, medical research databases, social work information, and the listings for CME and CEU opportunities

(*continued*)

Table 7.1

Examples of Databases (*continued*)

Database	Description
OVID, operated by the Wolters Kluwer Health publishing company, is internationally supported ■ Includes full bibliographical references, abstracts, full-text links, authors' full name references, other articles citing the article found ■ A paid subscription is needed to use this database, although many hospitals/institutions have access to OVID ■ Search aids are suggested on the screen ■ Education support and tutorials are available free of charge ■ Available in multiple languages	Key subject areas include agricultural and food sciences, bioengineering and biotechnology, clinical medicine, computer science and technology, dentistry, earth and environmental sciences, evidence-based medicine, geology and life sciences, neurology and neurosciences, nursing and allied health, pharmacy, philosophy and religion, physics, psychology and psychiatry, social sciences and the humanities, technical science, veterinary medicine, and zoology
PubMed was developed by the National Center for Biotechnology Information (NCBI) at the National Library of Medicine (NLM), located at the U.S. National Institutes of Health (NIH) ■ Publishers participating in PubMed electronically submit citations to NCBI before or at the time of publication ■ If the publisher has a website that offers full text of its journals, PubMed provides links to that site as well as biological resources, consumer health information, research tools, and more; however, there may be a charge to access the text or information ■ PubMed Tools: Used for clinical queries	Comprises more than 28 million citations for biomedical literature from MEDLINE, life science journals, and online books; citations may include links to full-text content from PubMed Central and publisher websites Allows the user to make clinical queries, match citations, and download Pubmed Mobile on your phone for easy access
MEDLINE (Medical Literature Analysis and Retrieval System Online; 1966–present) ■ Includes article full citation ■ Provides links to many (but not all) full-text articles and other related resources ■ The largest component of PubMed ■ A free accessible online database of biomedical journal citations and abstracts created by the U.S. NLM ■ Contains more than 5,200 journals published in the United States and more than 80 other countries that are currently indexed for MEDLINE ■ Available from the NLM homepage and can be searched for free at www.nlm.nih.gov	Studies in medicine, nursing, dentistry, psychiatry, veterinary medicine, and pharmacology

(*continued*)

Table 7.1

Database	Description
ERIC (Education Resources Information Center Institute of Education Sciences; 1966–present), an index of education journals ■ Contains more than 1.3 million bibliographical records of journal articles; most are peer reviewed ■ Abstracts and links to full text in .pdf format are available from individuals and publishers who give free full text; websites and libraries that may have full text are provided ■ For most materials from 2004 forward, if full text is not available in ERIC, links to publishers are provided ■ Contains journal articles, books, research synthesis, conference papers, technical reports, policy papers, and other education-related materials	Studies from the world of education; ERIC indexes materials from scholarly organizations, professional associations, research centers, policy organizations, university presses, the U.S. Department of Education, and other federal, state, and local agencies; individual contributors submit conference proceedings and papers, research papers, dissertations, and theses
Proquest Founded as a microfilm publisher, it began publishing doctoral dissertations in 1939. It has published more than 3 million searchable dissertations and thesis. It is the designated offsite digital archive for the U.S. Library of Congress	Contains dissertations and theses, primary source material, ebooks, scholarly journals, historical and current newspapers and periodicals, data sources, and other content of interest to a researcher
PsycINFO (corresponds to the print *Psychological Abstracts*; 1887–present) ■ Abstract database prepared by the American Psychological Association (APA) ■ Contains more than 2 million records selected from more than 2,000 journals ■ Also contains bibliographical citations, abstracts, cited references, and descriptive information across a wide variety of scholarly publications in the behavioral and social sciences ■ Available at www.apa.org/psycinfo	Studies from psychology and related disciplines; usually accessed through a vendor like OVID or APA
Cochrane Database of Systematic Reviews ■ Excellent source for "evidence" in evidence-based practice ■ Includes full text of reviews ■ Abstracts of reviews are available at https://www.cochranelibrary.com/cdsr/reviews	Full text of systematic reviews prepared by the Cochrane Collaboration, including completed reviews and protocols

CEU, continuing education unit; CME, continuing medical education.

- **ClinicalKey:** This database is a medical search engine and database tool owned by the medical and scientific publishing company Elsevier. They offer access to the medical library published by them.

ClinicalKey includes full-text articles from medical journals and medical reference books across a wide range of specialties. It contains clinically relevant drug information and more than 15,000 patient handouts and patient education guidelines. It answers questions quickly because it "thinks" like you do, recognizing relevant clinical concepts as you type and offering shortcuts to critical answers. It keeps you moving by bringing the most clinically relevant content to the top of your results page. It is available at www.clinicalkey.com/#!.

Full-Text Databases

When searching for research articles, look for sources that offer the full text of each article, including graphs, charts, and other illustrations. Vendors such as OVID include hyperlinks to references of full-text articles. The full-text article may be available in .pdf or .html format. Fewer vendors offer access to full-text medical books. Although online access to full-text medical books is growing, such access is still quite limited for nursing and allied health books.

Fast Facts

A hyperlink lets you click on a web address that automatically connects (or links) you to relevant material. Hyperlinks usually appear in bold type, underlined, or in a different color from the rest of the text.

Key Word Search

Most electronic databases require that you begin a search by identifying key words. Key words are terms that describe your subject of interest. For example, when searching for information about incarcerated women with HIV, you could use the key words *incarcerated women*, *HIV in prison*, *HIV in prisoners*, *prisoners with HIV*, or *AIDS in women*. Trying each of these key words will demonstrate how the manipulation of a few words can yield different lists of research articles.

Search Engines

A search engine is an information retrieval system stored on a computer system, such as the World Wide Web. One of the most popular search engines is Google, which was started in 1998.

Other search engines include:

- Bing
- Yahoo! Search
- Ask.com
- InfoSpace
- **DuckDuckGo** (emphasizes protecting searchers' privacy and avoiding the filter bubble of personalized search results)
- **SlideShare** (allows you to search for documented slideshow presentations)

The key to finding scholarly research articles is to use a search engine that yields reliable information. One free source that fits this requirement is Google Scholar (https://scholar.google.com/), which can be used to locate nursing research articles. It also indexes other resources that house inaccurate information and are not part of scholarly studies, such as:

- Commercial websites
- Individual home pages
- Advocacy websites
- Cheaters' websites

Remember that unlike scientific and scholarly literature and databases, Google is unfiltered, so the user should be very careful to evaluate the results provided through its searches. See Table 7.2 for the pros and cons of using Google Scholar. If you choose to use Google Scholar, you will find the following sources:

- Journal articles and abstracts from:
  - Publishers' websites (e.g., JSTOR, Muse, Wiley)
  - Free online databases (e.g., PubMed, ERIC)
  - Online journal websites (both free and subscription based)
- Peer-reviewed papers
- Selected books from:
  - Google book search
  - Open WorldCat

Google Scholar is not currently a comprehensive source for serious research, but it continues to grow and improve (see Table 7.2). Many students use it because it provides free access, and nurse

Table 7.2

Pros and Cons of Google Scholar	
Pros	**Cons**
■ Cross-disciplinary	■ Lacks advanced search features
■ Subjects do not neatly fit into one category	■ No stated editorial policy
	■ No controlled vocabulary
■ Includes both book and journal literature	■ Lacks standards for names
	■ Inconsistent coverage
■ Cited reference searching	■ Indexing reportedly lags PubMed by months
■ Citation checking	

scholars and other researchers increasingly are citing it. Occasionally, Google Scholar covers the nursing literature better than traditional databases. So, indeed, use it as a search engine if you want to be comprehensive, but use it in addition to CINAHL, MEDLINE, and other more traditional health information search engines. It may be helpful for topics that cross disciplinary boundaries.

CONDUCTING A BASIC LITERATURE SEARCH

Starting the Search

Now that you have accessed a database, how do you conduct the actual search? It is important to understand some terms that will assist in the search. To start a search on pediatric burn care, for example, access the computer's search engine, and enter the word *burns* in the search box as your **key word**, the word you choose for your search that describes your topic of interest.

Fast Facts

Remember that certain diseases can be known by different terms, so you need to search all of them to get a complete list of the relevant literature.

Example: SUBJECT HEADING: CEREBRAL VASCULAR ACCIDENT
Cerebral vascular accident can also be known as:
■ Stroke
■ CVA
■ Cerebrovascular accident

(continued)

(continued)

- Cerebral vascular accidents
- Cerebrovascular accidents
- CVAs
- Strokes

The CINAHL database is used in this instructional example. You can access this database on your computer at health.ebsco .com/products/cinahl-plus-with-full-text and follow along with the following search.

The Initial Search

After entering the term *burns* into the search window, the resulting search yields **8,170** journal articles. It is clear by this large number of articles that this search term was too broad. The next step is to refine the search by combining two key words from your topic of interest: *pediatrics* and *burns*. By inserting the word ***and*** as your **operator** between the key terms, the two terms will be connected, and the search will be more clearly defined. (The words *and*, *or*, and *not* are known as Boolean search operators; their use in refining searches is described later in this chapter.) Entering the refined search term *burns and pediatrics* now yields articles that contain both terms. The results have now identified 91 journal articles related to *burns and pediatrics*. Sometimes using these words can limit your search too much, so simply remove them and search again.

Stop Word

A stop word is a word that a search engine ignores when you conduct a query because the word is so common that it does not contribute to the relevancy of the search. Examples of these words are *and*, *get*, *the*, and *you* (Joos, Nelson, & Smith, 2014).

Narrowing the Search

Narrowing the search by using two key words produced results that more exactly apply to the topic in which you are interested. The search has narrowed the results to **91** articles that relate specifically to pediatric burns.

To narrow the search even further, you can put quotation marks around the words used as your key terms. Doing this will yield only titles that contain both your key search words. See the following section on quotation marks for more about using quotation marks when searching, or add more key words to refine your search even further.

Note that conducting a search using key word(s) is just one of many approaches. Searches also can be conducted using author name, article title, or journal title. Other options include basic searches, advanced searches, and searches that look for a specific citation in the text of an article. Simply select the method you want to use in conducting the search.

It is preferable to obtain articles that have full text so you will be able to read them. To determine which articles are available as full-text articles, do either of the following:

1. Scroll through all the results to look for those identified as "full-text" articles.
2. When conducting the search, click "Linked Full Text" in the "Limit Your Results" box on the right side of the screen.

Narrowing the search using a timeline is also possible. The CINAHL database includes a timeline in the box on the side of the screen, showing the years for which journal articles are available. To refine the search to reflect certain years, click "Update Results."

After updating, the search results list only seven articles that have full text. These full-text articles are available as .pdf files, .html files, or linked files. Click on the desired text format to obtain the full text of the selected journal article. Also note that the timeline has also narrowed to the years 1999 to 2007 from the broader timeline previously displayed.

Expanding the Search

Truncation

If, in contrast to the preceding example, the search using a key word produced only one hit, or result, the search would need to be expanded. To expand a search, you can enter the key word and then use the term *or* and truncation to increase your results. **Truncation is a technique that is used to find variant word endings**, as illustrated in the following examples:

Key Term	=	Truncations
Child*	=	child, children, children
Parent*	=	parent, parents, parenting
Spouse*	=	spouse, spouses, spousal

The truncation symbol varies by search engine, with *, !, ?, $, and # commonly used. For example:

Search Engine	Truncation Symbol to Use
EBSCOhost (CINAHL), ProQuest, others	*
OVID and MEDLINE	$
Google, Yahoo	automatic

To expand your search using the CINAHL database truncation symbol (*), enter the word followed by the symbol, as follows: *burns**. This will expand the search to include any articles that contain the word *burns* anywhere in the citation. Note that using the search term *burns** could produce articles written by an author named Burns, articles that include the word *burns* in the title of the article, or articles that simply mention *burns* once in the text.

Be aware that different key words can generate dramatically different results. For example, if the word *children* is substituted for the word *pediatrics*, the search yields only two results, and they are not even full-text articles. Do not become frustrated when this occurs. Conducting a search takes time. Be creative, "free think," and search using a variety of terms to experience how different search results can be.

Use of Other Terms to Expand or Narrow Your Search

Boolean Search Operators

Boolean logic defines logical relationships between terms in a search (Figure 7.1). The Boolean search operators are **and**, **or**, and **not**. When executing a search, *and* takes precedence over *or*.

- *And* combines search terms so that the text of each search result contains all of the terms. For example, **burns and pediatrics** finds articles that contain both *burns* and *pediatrics*.
- *Or* combines search terms so that each search result contains at least one of the terms. For example, **burn or pediatrics** finds results that contain either *burn* or *pediatrics*.
- *Not* excludes terms so that each search result does not contain any of the terms that follow it. For example, **television not cable** finds results that contain *television* but not *cable* (EBSCO Support, 2015).

Explode/Expand

You can also click to expand the subject heading, referred to as *exploding the heading*. The headings are exploded, or expanded, to

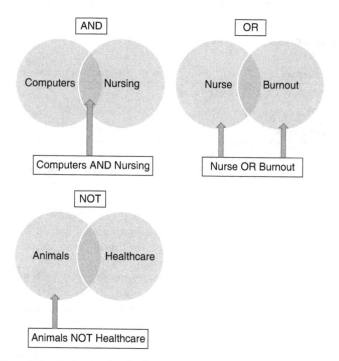

Figure 7.1 Understanding Boolean search strategies.
Source: Adapted from Joos, I., Nelson, R., & Smith, M. (2014). *Introduction to computers for healthcare professionals* (6th ed.). Boston, MA: Jones & Bartlett.

retrieve all references indexed to that term as well as all references indexed to any narrower subject terms. In this example, only "Burns, Inhalation" can be exploded. To explode these terms, check the box "Explode," and click on "Smoke Inhalation." In a database with a "tree" format, such as MeSH (Medical Subject Headings) or CINAHL, exploding retrieves all documents containing any of the subject terms below the term you selected. In other databases, exploding retrieves all documents containing the selected term as well as any of its first level of narrower terms. If a plus sign (+) appears next to a narrower or related term, there are narrower terms below it. Scan the list for a relevant term, and click in its checkbox. Then click "Continue." You will then find articles related to those subheadings.

Major Concept

If you want to search by major subject heading, select "Major Concept." This creates a search that finds only records for which the subject heading is a major point of the article. Searches are limited with specific qualifiers (subheadings) to improve the precision of the search. Major subject headings indicate the main concept of an article. Note that you can **use both explode and major concept at the same time** to retrieve references indexed to your term (and its narrower terms) and all articles for which the subject heading is the major point of the article (EBSCO Support, 2015).

Scope Notes

In some databases (e.g., CINAHL, MEDLINE), you can click on the word *scope* or the scope icon. This enables you to view the entire scope note, which is an explanation of a term and its synonyms.

Fast Facts

To focus your search on specific terms, try putting quotation marks around the word(s).

Using Quotation Marks When Searching

To narrow your search when using a database or search engine, **place quotation marks around the terms for your search**. The search will then yield only results that contain all of the words in your search term or phrase. If quotation marks are not used, the results will include references containing any of the words. Narrowing the search to the exact terms will make the search more successful in producing articles that reflect the topic of your research.

For example, suppose you enter the search term *"adult day cares"* as shown here, using quotation marks. The following article will appear. Note that the citation contains all three words.

1. *Adult day cares and public policy: a strategic plan for the Louisville metropolitan area.* Wishnia GS; Kentucky Nurse, 1997 Oct-Dec; 45 (4): 5

If you enter *adult day cares* without quotation marks, your search also will yield articles with any one of the words in them, as seen in the following three listings:

1. *Causation and intent: persistent conundrums in end-of-life care.* Rich BA; Cambridge Quarterly of Healthcare Ethics, 2007 Winter; 16 (1): 63–73
2. *Fostering the transition from pediatric to adult neurosurgical care.* Abraham S; AXON/L'AXONE, 2007 Winter; 28 (2): 13

3. *What kills one woman every minute of every day?* Kantrowitz B; Newsweek, 2007 Jul 2–9; 150 (2): 56, 57

Searching by Publication or Journal

If the search produces a reference or citation to a journal article that you would like to use, locate the journal in a database by searching for the name of the publication or journal. To do this, click on the publication tab, and search alphabetically by the first letter of the name of the journal to see if the database has your journal.

PROVIDERS OF RESEARCH DATABASES

EBSCOhost

EBSCOhost is an online source for the e-journals available at your library. With EBSCOhost, you can:

- **Find a specific journal** quickly by using the Find Journals feature.
- **Browse through a list of all journals** available with the Browse feature.
- Browse a list of **subject categories**, then view a list of all journals that fall in a category of interest. This allows you to easily find journals that cover specific topics.
- **Find specific articles** quickly using the Find Articles feature. Search by the article title or by the author's name.
- **Find articles that cover a specific topic** by searching for key words in the titles, abstracts, and even full text of millions of articles.
- Read article abstracts, and **link directly to the full text** of the articles you find.

An example of a citation you may find in EBSCOhost is:

Hepatitis A seroprevalence and risk factors among day-care educators. (includes abstract) Muecke CJ; Clinical & Investigative Medicine, 2004 Oct; 27 (5): 259–64 (journal article research, tables/charts) PMID: 15559862 CINAHL AN: 2005114261
PDF Full Text HTML Full Text Linked Full Text

You can then click on "PDF Full Text" and receive the full text article in a .pdf format. Or you can opt to receive the full-text article in an .html file. Clicking on the "Linked Full Text" tab will hyper-link you to a site where you can access full text or may automatically download the full-text format for you.

OVID Online

OVID, operated by Wolters Kluwer Health, provides information for professionals and students in medicine, nursing, allied health, pharmacy, and the pharmaceutical industry. It consists of hundreds of databases, including more than 1,200 journals and books from dozens of publishers. OVID offers training programs to assist users with their searches. More information about OVID can be found in Table 7.1 and online at www.ovid.com/site. Another online tutorial for OVID is available at www.ovid.com/site/support/training.jsp.

Using the OVID Database

As with any search, you need to begin with a search term. In the example below, *geriatrics* is the search term. A search using this term would yield the following response, indicating that 5,456 results have been matched to your term:

Results of your search: geriatrics.mp. [mp=title, abstract, full text, caption text]
Viewing 1–10 of 5456 Results

That is a lot of articles to look through. Listed as number 14, below, is one result, with its reference information. Somewhere in this article, geriatrics is mentioned. As you can see, this search yields results that are quite broad and may not be exactly what you are looking for.

14. U.S. Preventive Services Task Force. Screening for Chlamydial Infection: U.S. Preventive Services Task Force Recommendation Statement. Annals of Internal Medicine. 147(2):128–134, July 17, 2007.

So, you might want to refine your search by adding another search term. Perhaps *"geriatrics and stroke"* might yield more specific results. To the right of the citation on the OVID screen is a list of options:

- Complete Reference
- Table of Contents
- OVID Full Text
- Full Text
- Abstract

Click on the one that best fulfills your needs. Complete Reference will give you just that—a complete reference of the article. Table of Contents will give you the contents of a book or periodical. OVID Full Text will give you the full text with the journal name at the top of the article. Full Text will give you the full text of the article with the database name on the top of it. If you want just the abstract, click on that to receive the specific information you want.

PubMed

PubMed Central (PMC) is the free digital archive of biomedical and life sciences journal literature at the U.S. NIH's National Library of Medicine (NLM). It includes more than 24 million citations from MEDLINE and other life science and biomedical journal articles dating back to the 1950s. PubMed provides links to full-text articles and other related resources as well as online books. All the articles in PMC are free (sometimes on a delayed basis), as is access to available abstracts. More information about PubMed can be found at www .ncbi.nlm.nih.gov/pmc.

Journals and Magazines

When you are searching for journal articles, be sure to use only research articles published in scholarly journals. Keep in mind that articles in magazines and some journals may not be written by a researcher or even by an expert in the field or a member of the medical profession. In such cases, you are actually reading someone else's opinion about the research; this is sometimes, but not always, presented in an editorial format. Therefore, it is important to look at both the author and the source of the information you are using. You should read research articles written by a researcher or an expert in your area of interest. Table 7.3 lists several differences between magazines and scholarly journals.

It is also important to pay attention to the type of journal. The field of nursing has many nursing journals, available online or in print format. For many specialties, such as pediatrics, you will find many relevant journals whose articles are written by physicians, nurses, scientists, editors, and other professionals. Look at the journal to see if it offers research findings or just informational articles about a particular disease process or clinical application. Although these may be very important, they do not lead to compelling evidence in EBP. If you recall the hierarchy of strong evidence, research from randomized controlled trials is the strongest evidence. You will not find that in journals that offer information-type articles. So you will need to look to a scholarly journal that includes only peer-reviewed articles. More information about this type of journal is provided in the following text and in Table 7.3.

Table 7.3

Differences Between Magazines and Scholarly Journals

	Magazines	Scholarly Journals
Author	Journalist; layperson; sometimes unknown; may be scholar, but not necessarily in the field covered	Identified expert, scholar, or professor in the field
Notes	Few or no references or notes	Includes notes or bibliography, or both
Style	Journalistic; written for average reader	Written for experts; shows research
Editing	Reviewed by one or more people employed by the magazine	Editorial board of outside scholars reviews articles before they are accepted for publication
Audience	General public	Scholars or researchers in the field
Look	Glossy; many pictures, often in color	More sedate look, mostly print
Frequency	Usually weekly or monthly	Usually quarterly or monthly
Contents	Current events; general interest	More specialized; research topics
Indexes	Found in general periodical indexes (e.g., Reader's Guide)	Found in subject-specialized indexes

Source: Adapted from https://www.library.georgetown.edu/tutorials/scholarly-vs-popular

Online Journals

A large number of journals are now available online. These journals may be referred to as **e-journals** or **e-zines.** At www.nursingcenter.com, operated by Wolters Kluwer Health, you can view the contents of the most current issue of more than 50 leading journals. You can also go directly to each journal's home page, where you can usually view the most current issue of the journal. If you are looking for a pediatric journal, for example, you can enter *pediatric nursing journals* into any search engine, such as Google, and a multitude of

Table 7.4

Free Online Nursing Journals	
Journal	**URL**
Allnurses.com (web journal about critical care and emergency nursing)	www.allnurses.com
Imprint (magazine for nursing students) from the National Student Nurses Association (NSA)	www.nsna.org
Internet Scientific Publications	www.ispub.com
Nursing World	www.nursingworld.org
Online Journal of Issues in Nursing	www.nursingcenter.com
Journal Informatics Nursing	www.ania.org/publications/journal

journals will pop up. If you are interested in geriatric journals, you can enter *geriatrics*, and similar results for geriatric journal websites will appear. Table 7.4 lists some of the nursing journals that can be accessed for free online.

Evidence-Based Practice Center

Another great place to search, especially if you are looking for eidence beyond that provided through the Cochrane Collaboration, is the AHRQ. Its EBPC provides reports that are used for informing and developing coverage decisions, quality measures, educational materials and tools, guidelines, and research agendas. For more information on the EBPC, including a list of archived reports, visit the AHRQ website (www.guideline.gov/resources/ahrq-evidence-reports.aspx). In addition, if you do an Internet search for *evidence-based practice guidelines*, you will find that many disciplines, such as orthopedics, have websites that are designated to best practice in their particular specialty area.

Scholarly Journals and Peer-Reviewed Journals or Articles

Scholarly Journals

A scholarly journal contains articles written by scholars, researchers, professors, or experts in the field on topics related to that journal. The journal has a review process in place, and less emphasis is placed on advertising. It usually includes research articles that are of interest to other professionals in that field (see Table 7.3).

BOX 7.1 SCHOLARLY NURSING JOURNALS FOR RESEARCH

Advances in Nursing Science
American Journal of Nursing
Canadian Journal of Nursing Research
Clinical Nursing Research
Dimensions of Critical Care Nursing
Evidence-Based Nursing
International Journal of Nursing Studies
Journal of Advanced Nursing
Journal of Nursing Scholarship
Journal of Research in Nursing
Nurse Researcher
Nursing Research
Nursing Science Quarterly
Research and Theory for Nursing Practice
Western Journal of Nursing Research

Peer-Reviewed Articles

If an article is peer reviewed, it means that it has been read and approved for publication by experts in the field of the research topic. Usually, more than one reviewer's approval is required for publication. The review process is usually blinded, which means that the reviewers do not know the name of the author so that personal relationships do not enter the process. All identifying author criteria and credentials are omitted from the article prior to the review process.

Box 7.1 lists a sampling of scholarly journals that you might want to consult in your search for research journals appropriate to your topic of interest.

Grey Literature

Grey literature includes works that may not have been formally peer reviewed and may not have appeared in standard or recognized journals, publications, or databases. Government agencies, universities, corporations, associations and societies, research centers, and professional organizations produce this type of literature. For example, some nursing e-magazines appear on the Internet as a credible source, but have not been subject to peer or scholarly review. These do not have a wide distribution, but they do appear on the Internet within the domain of healthcare information (Joos et al., 2014).

Fast Facts

Now that you have found a research article, how do you know it is a good one? Remember the principles you learned in Chapters 5, Quantitative Research, and 6, Qualitative Research, as part of quantitative and qualitative research design. Make sure the articles are relevant, and follow the sound principles of research. Evaluate the evidence. We explore this step in the next chapter.

REFERENCES

EBSCO Support. (2015). *Searching with Boolean operators—Help sheet.* Retrieved from https://www.epsnj.org/site/handlers/filedownload.ash x?moduleinstanceid=7675&dataid=31759&FileName=searching%20 tips%20EBSCO.pdf

Joos, I., Nelson, R., & Smith, M. (2014). *Introduction to computers for healthcare professionals* (6th ed.). Boston, MA: Jones & Bartlett.

8

Evaluating the Evidence

Now that you have found your research article, how do you know if it is a good article or a flawed one? When doing an evidence-based practice (EBP) project, it is very important that you use reliable evidence. You would not want to recommend a change to a clinical practice based on evidence that is not "good" or on the basis of one study. This chapter discusses how to evaluate the evidence that you have found in order to design your EBP proposal.

In this chapter, you will learn:

1. How to evaluate the evidence you found by asking five key questions
2. How to critique research articles using a simple worksheet provided in the chapter appendix
3. How to use the rating hierarchy to evaluate the evidence

TIME TO EVALUATE THE EVIDENCE

Now that you have found evidence, you need to determine if the evidence is good enough to warrant a recommendation to suggest a change in practice. It is essential that the evidence be carefully scrutinized. You would not want to propose a change in practice based on flawed or biased information.

To determine if a study is relevant to your EBP project, you will need practice in analyzing the research. You may want to consult a research text for a more detailed understanding of this process. This chapter briefly discusses how to analyze evidence. Remember that just because a research study is published in a peer-reviewed journal does not ensure that it was well designed or well conducted. It does not guarantee that data were accurately analyzed or accurately reported in the publication. You need to think about how the study was designed, how the research was carried out, and how the data were analyzed. If a tool was used in the study, was it tested prior to use and proved to be both reliable and valid? Some general questions you may want to ask when examining studies are listed in Box 8.1. Also review Table 5.2 in Chapter 5, Quantitative Research, and Table 6.2 in Chapter 6, Qualitative Research, which offer guides to critiquing quantitative and qualitative research. Figure 8.1 provides a schematic illustration of an evidence hierarchy that can assist you in determining the levels of the evidence, or the strength of the evidence, in a study. As an alternative to the Melnyk and Fineout-Overholt method (see data presented in Chapter 1, Introduction to Evidence-Based Practice, Box 1.2), there is the Johns Hopkins Nursing Quality of Evidence Appraisal (see Table 8.1). You might find this useful in gaining understanding of evaluating evidence.

Fast Facts

Never suggest or recommend changing practice on the basis of one research study. Many novices who embark on an EBP project are so happy to find one study on their topic of interest that they base their entire project on it. This should never be done.

As you begin to analyze the evidence for your EBP project, you need to ask yourself five key questions about the research study you are evaluating:

1. What were the results of the study?
2. Are the results valid?
3. Are the results reliable?
4. Will the results help me provide improved care for my patients?
5. Do the results make sense for my patient population?

Let's take a look at each of these questions more closely.

BOX 8.1 SOME BASIC QUESTIONS TO ASK WHEN EVALUATING RESEARCH EVIDENCE

- Is the research study relevant or important to nursing?
- Is the abstract present, and does it include the purpose, method, and summary of findings of the study?
- Was a theoretical or philosophical framework used for the study?
- Is there a hypothesis?
- How many subjects (or participants) were there?
- Was the number of subjects (or participants) relevant for the type of study done?
- How were the subjects (or participants) selected?
- What method of data collection was used?
- Was the data collection method sound and accurate?
- Did the data collection method provide reliable and valid results?
- How were the data analyzed, and was this method appropriate for the study?
- Are any assumptions for the study included?
- Are limitations of the study included?
- Are suggestions for future research included?
- Is there a discussion of the results?
- Is any bias revealed in the data?
- Is there any researcher bias? For example, was the study done using students from a college where the researcher works? Does the study recommend a medication when funds to conduct the research were provided by the manufacturer of the medication?
- Were any ethical situations discussed, or were any ethical procedures violated?
- Did the authors obtain institutional review board (IRB) approval and informed consent prior to the start of the study?

What Were the Results of the Study?

What exactly are the results of the study? Do they make sense and answer the research question(s)? For example, in a quantitative interventional study, how significant are the treatment effects? Is there a significant difference between the patients who received the intervention and those who did not? If not, then the study does not prove the intervention is successful, and no practice change should be recommended based on these results. In a qualitative study, did the research approach fit the purpose of the study? Was it congruent? In other words, did the results of the study make sense and answer the research questions? The results should be a logical explanation of the intent of the research project and should not be erroneous or answer a question other than the research questions. For example, if the researchers were looking at the effect of a nursing intervention in the lived experience of parents of children with a chronic illness, what common threads or themes were found? Do they make sense? Do they fit in the context of the situation or living environment? Did the nursing intervention make a difference or not? If it did not, there would be no need to employ that intervention in your practice. If it did make a difference and the researcher is telling you that it did, examine this intervention further to determine if it might work with your patient population or in your situation.

Are the Results Valid?

Validity means that the results measure what they were supposed to measure. For example, in an experimental or interventional study,

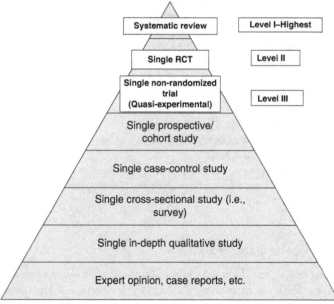

Figure 8.1 Schematic of evidence hierarchy.
RCT, randomized controlled trial.
Source: Adapted from Polit, D. G., & Beck, C. T. (2016). *Nursing research: Generating and assessing evidence for nursing practice* (10th ed.). Philadelphia, PA: Wolters Kluwer.

Table 8.1

Johns Hopkins Nursing Quality of Evidence Appraisal

Grade	Nomenclature	Definition for Research Evidence	Definition for Nonresearch Evidence
A	High	Consistent results, sufficient sample size, adequate control, and definitive conclusions; consistent recommendations based on extensive literature review that includes thoughtful reference to scientific evidence	Expertise is clearly evident
B	Good	Reasonably consistent results, sufficient sample size, some control, and fairly definitive conclusions; reasonably consistent recommendations based on fairly comprehensive literature review that includes some reference to scientific evidence	Expertise appears to be credible
C	Low/Major Flaw	Little evidence with inconsistent results, insufficient sample size, conclusions cannot be drawn	Expertise is not discernable or is dubious

Source: Newhouse, R. P., Dearholt, S., Poe, S., Pugh, L., White, K. (2007). *Johns Hopkins nursing evidence-based practice: Model and guidelines* (p. 207). Indianapolis, IN: Sigma Theta Tau International.

were the participants or subjects randomly assigned to control, treatment, or intervention groups? Were they equal with respect to key characteristics prior to the study? Were intervening or extraneous variables controlled? Suppose the research study measured whether taking acetaminophen (Tylenol) every 4 hours around the clock would keep a child from getting a fever. Did the results show the child was fever free, or did the child develop a fever? If the results showed the child subsequently had a fever, then the research study (to take acetaminophen every 4 hours around the clock as a fever preventive) did not prove the hypothesis. Thus, you would not want to develop a protocol stating that administering acetaminophen every 4 hours around the clock will prevent a child's fever.

Are the Results Reliable?

Does the research study measure what it is supposed to measure on subsequent experiences? Consider the previous example involving acetaminophen. If the research study reported that giving acetaminophen every 4 hours alleviated (rather than prevented) fever, did this happen just one time, or did it happen consistently for all subjects in the research study? Suppose there were two studies, with varying or contradictory results. If one research study showed that giving acetaminophen every 4 hours around the clock alleviated fever and another study showed that it did not, the second study negates the findings of the first study, and the study results are not conclusive. So based on these two research studies, a practice change should not be implemented.

Will the Results Help Me Provide Improved Care for My Patients?

Were the subjects or participants in the research study similar to the patients of interest in your EBP project? Are the benefits of the intervention or treatment greater than the inherent risks? Will implementation of these results make a difference in caring for your patients? Let's say that you work with adult patients. Can the results of the pediatric study with acetaminophen be applied to adult patients? No, they cannot. If you are a pediatric nurse, will the differing results of the two studies described earlier help you in caring for children? No, because the two studies contradict each other. Are the benefits of giving acetaminophen every 4 hours (the intervention) greater than the inherent risk? Suppose you were to give acetaminophen every 4 hours around the clock for several days. Although it might (or might not) help control a child's fever, could it cause liver damage? In September 2002, the Food and Drug Administration (FDA) Nonprescription Advisory Board reported that acetaminophen can cause liver damage and failure. Therefore, no one should take more than the recommended dosage and the drug should not be taken for more than 4 days (United States Food and Drug Administration, 2018). The evidence indicates that overusing acetaminophen (accidentally or intentionally) is the leading cause of liver failure in the United States (Fontana, 2008). This is a simple example of how research and finding evidence can impact nursing practice.

Do the Results Make Sense for My Patient Population?

If you find the results of a research study far-fetched and vastly opposed to your experience and current practice, read it with caution. You do not need to include every research study on a topic as evidence in your EBP project. This is particularly so if the study population, setting, or other key parameters of the study do not match those of the setting where your EBP project would be implemented. Always ask yourself, "Does this make sense?"

These are some basic questions to ask when looking at the results of a research study. Now, let's look more closely at the actual components of the research study report. A simple worksheet can be used for this purpose (see Appendix 8.1). The sections that follow break down each component addressed on the worksheet.

KEY AREAS TO EXAMINE WHEN CRITIQUING A RESEARCH STUDY ARTICLE

Type of Study

What Type of Study Is the Research Article?

Is it quantitative or qualitative?

Author Qualifications

What are the qualifications of the person who did the research? Is the person qualified to do the study? For example, if you are evaluating a research article on children's pain levels and the researcher never worked with children and does not routinely assess pain in practice, he or she would not be qualified. Similarly, suppose you are evaluating a research article looking at education of student nurses. It would make sense if the researcher were a professor or someone who understands and works with nursing students.

Title

Does the title describe what the research study is about? Is the title short and concise or long and convoluted? For example, let's say you are interested in children's reactions to stress in the hospital. The title of an article you have located is "How Do Adults Respond to Stress?" This article would not be appropriate for your EBP project because it does not mention the patient population that is the focus of your study (i.e., children).

Abstract

The abstract is the summary of all points of the research study. It should contain enough information to enable you to evaluate key aspects of the study. The abstract should contain the **purpose, research question(s), method**, and **major findings** of the study. Does it contain these items, and does it summarize the results of the study? What is the exact method or process the researcher(s) used in conducting the study? How was the study done? Is the topic interesting and relevant to your patient population or the problem of interest for your EBP project?

Introduction

An introductory paragraph should always be included. This paragraph should not only present the topic, but also grab your interest and provide a brief overview of the topic at hand. What is the research problem? Basically, what is the point of the study? Has the researcher appropriately described the scope of the problem? Does the problem have significance for the nursing profession? How will the research contribute to nursing practice, nursing administration, or nursing education? Is the problem to be addressed formally presented as a statement of purpose, research question, or hypothesis to be tested? Is this information communicated clearly and concisely?

Purpose

The purpose of the study should always be stated. It is very important to understand the motivation of researchers and how they feel their research study will advance either nursing science or nursing care. If it is a not a nursing-based study, the researcher should still explain what purpose the study hopes to serve in the healthcare environment.

Research Questions

Every research study should have a research question or questions as a guide. What question(s) does the researcher hope to answer? It is important to note that these questions are not the same thing as the purpose of the study. The research questions should fulfill the purpose, but they are not the same as the purpose.

Hypothesis

All quantitative research studies have a hypothesis or prediction of what the researcher thinks is going to happen. By developing a hypothesis, researchers are better able to identify possible sources of their own bias. Most often when researchers conduct research, they have a sense or indication of how the study will turn out. They may be trying to prove their hypothesis or prediction either correct or incorrect. This is an important part of the research study process. It is also important that the hypothesis makes sense for the study at hand. It would make no sense to make a prediction that cannot even be proved by the planned research study. If the report does not formally state any hypotheses, is the reason stated? Do the hypotheses (if any) flow from a theory or previous research? If not, what is the basis for the researcher's predictions? Are the hypotheses (if any) properly worded (i.e., do they state a predicted relationship between two or more variables)? Is there a rationale for the manner in which they were stated? Are hypotheses stated as research hypotheses or null hypotheses?

Fast Facts

Remember that qualitative studies do not have a hypothesis or test a hypothesis as do quantitative studies. In qualitative studies, the goal is to understand a phenomenon as it naturally exists in the world and to identify common themes. Predictions of outcome are not made. The qualitative researcher uses broad research questions to guide the study and seeks to understand meaningful patterns that evolve.

Literature Review

An extensive review of the literature should be completed. It is important to view all research done on a given topic before embarking on any future research. It is commonly said that we need to know where we've been to know where we are going or plan to go. The literature review should include relevant research studies, particularly those published within the past 5 years. If older studies are included, their importance should be explained. If they are landmark studies, propose significant changes, or reflect discoveries in the area being researched, include them. Confirm that the coverage of the literature seems thorough and complete. Does it appear that the review includes all or most of the major studies that have been conducted on the topic of interest? Are recent research reports cited? How recent are the reports? Does the review rely on appropriate materials (i.e., mainly on research reports, using primary or secondary sources)? Is the review organized so that development of ideas is clear? If the review is part of a research report for a new study, does the review support the need for the new research study? If the review is designed to guide clinical practice, does the review support the need for (or lack of need for) changes in practice? Does the review conclude with a synopsis of the state-of-the-art knowledge on the topic? Is the style of the review appropriate? Does the reviewer paraphrase, or is there an overreliance on quotations? Does the review appear unbiased? Does the reviewer use appropriate language? Does the review flow logically?

Fast Facts

Keep in mind that the length of time between the completion of a study and its publication in a scholarly journal may be up to 2 years. Therefore, many of the most recent research articles are already outdated before they are published. The time lag to publication varies from journal to journal.

Ethical Aspects of the Study

When examining a research study, you want to be sure the study was conducted ethically, especially if you plan to use it for evidence. No study participants should ever be subjected to physical harm, discomfort, or psychological distress. The researchers must take appropriate steps to keep them from being harmed. It is important when doing, and evaluating, research to consider whether the research benefit to participants in the study outweighs any potential risk to them. In addition, consider whether the benefits to society outweigh the costs to the participants. No type of coercion or undue influence should be used in recruiting or selecting the participants. When working with vulnerable subjects, special considerations need to be observed. The participants should never be deceived or tricked in any way to participate in the study. They must be made fully aware that they are participating in a study. It is the responsibility of researchers to ensure that the participants understand the purpose of the study and why the research is being done. Informed consent must always be obtained. Steps to ensure privacy and confidentiality must also be taken to protect the participants. Lastly, when a research study is conducted in an institution, such as a hospital, the research must be approved and monitored by an IRB or other similar ethics review committee.

Fast Facts

Vulnerable subjects are people who are not capable of giving a fully informed consent. This could be the result of mental incapacity or age. Examples of vulnerable subjects are children, mentally challenged or emotionally disabled people, someone in a coma, severely or terminally ill people, and pregnant women. Note that pregnant women can give informed consent, but the unborn fetus cannot. The risk to the unborn fetus must be examined, and the risk–benefit ratio for the pregnant mother and for the fetus must be weighed heavily when embarking on a research study. This is documented in the Code of Federal Regulations, 2005 (available online at www.hhs.gov/ohrp/policy/ohrpregulations.pdf).

Conceptual and Theoretical Frameworks

A conceptual or theoretical framework guides the study. Remember the framework does not have to come only from the field of nursing; it can be from another discipline, such as psychology (see Chapter 3, The Iowa Model of Evidence-Based Practice to Promote Quality

Care). But whatever framework is chosen, it should be relevant for the study. Does it flow? Does the framework make sense for the type of study? Is it explained clearly?

Operational Terms

Operational terms are terms that may have different meanings when used in different contexts. So the study should explain how such words will be defined. Do the researchers provide definitions of these terms and how each will be used in the study? If operational terms are used, are the terms and their definitions appropriate for the given study, and do they help to clarify exactly what each term means in the context of the study?

Research Design

What is the basic type of design? Remember that there are two main types of research: quantitative and qualitative. Within each of these categories, what type of design is used for the study? For example, is a quantitative study experimental or nonexperimental in design? Recall that in an experimental comparative or randomized study, the study participants are divided into two groups: experimental and control. The first group receives the experimental drug, therapy, treatment, or intervention, whereas the second group does not. Keep in mind that random assignment to these groups is necessary for experimental studies. If study participants are randomly assigned, the results are more credible and can be generalized to other similar studies (Carlson, Kruse, & Rouse, 1999). In addition, examine whether there are variables. If so, how do they affect each other? Identify the basic type of design to help your understanding of the content of the research. See Chapter 5, Quantitative Research, and Chapter 6, Qualitative Research, for further clarification of the different types of research designs. Always remember to check for bias in the study. Are any influences present that might have affected the results?

Fast Facts

The researcher should try to control threats to validity in any study. Validity is the ability to measure what is supposed to be measured. In research studies, an inference is made, or reasons or causes and a rationale are given describing the study results (the effect). When there are threats to validity, a study may contain incorrect inferences. Although it is hard to control every aspect or outcome of a study, the researcher must try to control as many variables as he or she can.

Population and Sample

How were the subjects or participants for the study selected? Was randomization used?

Quantitative Sampling Designs

Is the population identified, described, and easily accessible? Are eligibility criteria clearly described? Are the sample selection procedures clearly described? What type of sampling plan was used? Does the sample adequately represent the total population? Did some factor affect the representativeness of the sample (e.g., a low response rate)? Are possible sample biases identified? Is the sample size sufficiently large or too small?

Qualitative Sampling Designs

Is the setting adequately described? Are the setting and population appropriate for the research question(s)? How were the participants selected for the study? Was the sampling approach appropriate? Is the sample size adequate, too small, or too large? Did the researcher state that information saturation was achieved?

Data Collection Methods

Who collected the research data? Were the data collectors qualified for this role, or is there something about them (e.g., their professional role, their relationship with study participants) that could undermine the collection of unbiased, high-quality data? How were data collectors trained? Does the training appear adequate? Where and under what circumstances were the data gathered? Were other people present during the data collection? Could the presence of others have created any influence or bias? Did the collection of data place any undue burdens (in terms of time or stress) on participants? How might this have affected data quality?

Fast Facts

Interrater reliability is a term used when two or more individuals, or "coders," are gathering information during a study. It describes the degree to which they agree. For judging purposes, it is a consensus, that is, how often they agree on a given score. In research, it is how often two observers agree on a given item and the level of agreement between them. This level of agreement is very important in research when more than one person is gathering the data.

Statistical Significance

Were the collected data statistically significant? All the data in the world could be collected, but if they are not statistically significant, they are meaningless. It is very important to achieve statistical significance. The two easiest ways of understanding statistical significance are to look at the p value and the confidence interval. Review Chapter 5, Quantitative Research, for further explanation of these concepts.

Significance for Your Area of Practice

Most important when evaluating evidence is to ask yourself this question: Is this information significant to my patient population or EBP project? If it is not, then discard it; if it is, keep it for evidence.

Assumptions and Limitations

Assumptions are presuppositions that the researcher makes about the study before it begins. This is what the researcher is "taking for granted," so to speak. For example, the researcher may assume that people want to participate in the study.

Limitations prevent the study from reaching its full potential. An example would be if a researcher wanted to study the effects of sunshine on people's happiness, but it rained for the duration of the study. Another example would be if the researcher wanted to study 10-year-old boys, but only two 10-year-old boys were available. These limitations should be discussed and presented.

Conclusions

Do you agree with the conclusions the author or researcher drew from the study? In your opinion, did he or she draw incorrect conclusions or jump to conclusions not easily made from the evidence?

Implications for Future Research

Does the author or researcher explain the implications of the findings for future research? These are areas identified by the researcher for further exploration and research. Another researcher may choose to pursue these areas of research, but they also provide ideas for new or novice researchers embarking on a research project. Indeed, reviewing the research literature and current EBP guidelines may help you identify other areas in need of further practice changes for future research projects.

Summary

Ask yourself the basic questions in this section when reviewing evidence for your EBP project. The worksheet that accompanies this chapter (see Appendix 8.1) does not list all the questions that should be asked but gives the novice a good basis for evaluating research studies. In addition, you should review the guidelines for critiquing quantitative and qualitative studies provided in Chapter 5, Quantitative Research, and Chapter 6, Qualitative Research (see Tables 5.2 and 6.2).

In a research study, French (2006) found that specialist nurses use two main criteria, relevance and quality, to evaluate research in practice. Other criteria given in order of frequency were effectiveness, practicality, impact, effort, staff, and feasibility.

- *Effectiveness* meant whether the intervention was going to do what it intended to do.
- *Practicality* meant whether implementation of an intervention was functional, efficient, or sufficient in meeting the purpose for which it was intended.
- *Impact* described how the patient reacted to the intervention and whether the intervention could cause a patient any harm.
- *Effort* related to how easy it would be to implement the intervention.
- *Staff* referred to how nurses would be affected by implementing the intervention.
- *Feasibility* was the last and most consistent criterion examined: How difficult or feasible would it be to implement this nursing intervention?

You will probably relate to these criteria when examining evidence to determine whether to recommend implementation of an intervention in your practice area.

In a second study, Sandelowski and Barroso (2002) examined how to isolate the findings in qualitative research, as sometimes the data are misrepresented as findings. This means that some data are presented that may not be findings that relate to the study at hand. In addition, reports sometimes contain very little description to support the researcher's interpretations of the data. For example, how does the researcher eliminate his or her own biases in the interpretation of the data? Quotations and descriptions of incidents may be misused. Extensive quoting of participants may be included, but these quotations may not fit with the purpose of the study or the conclusions obtained, or they may be excessive in number. Researchers also sometimes do not state how they came up with patterns or themes. Finally, conceptual conclusions or theories that are used may drift from one concept to another and not truly represent the theory given as a basis for a study. These are some of the challenges highlighted by Sandelowski and Barroso (2002) in locating and evaluating the findings in qualitative research articles. So, if you become confused in determining what is good or bad research, do not hesitate to consult a person who has more experience in critiquing research. This can be a colleague, a professor at a local college, or someone in your institution's research department.

When rating evidence for EBP, the highest level of evidence is that obtained from a systematic review or meta-analysis of all relevant randomized controlled trials (RCTs) or established EBP clinical guidelines.

THE STRENGTH OF THE EVIDENCE

How strong is the evidence being used? What level of research is being used? There are numerous ways to grade or evaluate research evidence for use in EBP. The Agency for Healthcare Research and Quality (AHRQ) is a federally funded agency that supports quality of care and EBP through evidence-based practice centers (EBPCs) across the United States. The U.S. Preventive Services Task Force (USPSTF), which is supported by AHRQ, evaluates scientific studies related to clinical preventive services and makes recommendations based on specific criteria. These recommendations allow clinicians to make informed practice decisions. This task force grades the evidence using a letter system of A (strongly recommends), B (recommends), C (no recommendation for or against), D (recommends against), or I (insufficient evidence to recommend for or against). The evidence is graded on quality, quantity, and consistency (Long, 2009). More information about this system can be obtained at www.ahrq .gov/research/findings/final-reports/uspstf/uspstfeval.pdf.

The AHRQ recently supported a study in which 121 systems designed to rate evidence were evaluated to determine best practice in this area. The results identified gaps in rating quality, strength of evidence, and application of these grading schemes to the less traditional types of research, such as observational studies. The authors concluded that there is not (nor will there be in the near future) a single system that can be used to grade scholarly work across all disciplines. They also concluded that evidence gathering differs from clinician to clinician. These results show the difficulty in determining exactly what evidence is and how it might best be applied to practice (Malloch & Porter-O'Grady, 2005). For more information about this study and current recommendations, see www.ahrq.gov/Clinic/epcix.htm.

One of the most common evidence rating systems in nursing was put forth by Melnyk and Fineout-Overholt (2010) and consists of a seven-level hierarchy (see Box 1.2). Several other evidence ranking and grading schemes also exist, and controversy over which one is best led to an international effort to develop a universal system of evaluation. In 2000, an informal collaboration of people addressed the shortcomings and multiple evidence grading systems in healthcare. The international system that resulted is known by the acronym GRADE, which stands for grades of recommendation, assessment, development, and evaluation. The GRADE rating hierarchy offers another way to evaluate your evidence to see which of your research articles offers the strongest type of evidence available. It ranks evidence into four levels: (1) high, (2) moderate, (3) low, and (4) very low. The recommendation is either (1) strong or (2) weak (Long, 2009). You can learn more about the GRADE system at https://www .uptodate.com/home/grading-guide.

Sometimes it is helpful to have a tool to critique studies when you are first starting out. Please see Appendix 8.1 for an example of a tool you can use.

Fast Facts

Critiquing the evidence in a research study is a complex task and can be very confusing. You should know how to ask questions and review important aspects of the evidence and research reports you find. Understand how to grade the evidence and how to determine what makes evidence strong or weak. Efforts have been undertaken by various groups to develop a uniform system of evidence evaluation so that research is graded or evaluated in the same way.

APPENDIX 8.1

Article Critique Worksheet

When critiquing a research study article, answer the following questions by filling in the blank or circling your response.

1. Is the study **quantitative** or **qualitative**?
2. Is the **researcher qualified**? (yes or no) Why or why not?

_____

_____

_____

3. Is the **title** appropriate? (yes or no) Clear and concise? (yes or no)

4. **Abstract**
   - Is the hypothesis or research question present? (yes or no) If so, list it.

   _____

   _____

   _____

   - What is the method of research?

   _____

   _____

   _____

   - Is a description of the findings present? (yes or no)
   - Are the major findings listed? (yes or no) If so, what are they?

   _____

   _____

   _____

5. Introduction
   - Introductory paragraph? (yes or no)
   - Does the introduction grab your interest? (yes or no)
   - Any background information? (yes or no)
   - Is the significance to nursing stated? (yes or no)

6. What is the **purpose** of this research article?

   _____

   _____

   _____

7. Is the **research problem** identified? (yes or no) What is it?

   _____

   _____

   _____

8. **Hypothesis**
   - Is the hypothesis stated? (yes or no) What is it?

   _____

   _____

   _____

   - Do you think the hypothesis makes sense (is a good guess) for the given study? (yes or no) Why or why not?

   _____

   _____

   _____

9. **Literature review**
   - How many articles are reviewed by the author and listed in the reference section? _____
   - Is it an adequate number in your opinion? (yes or no)
   - Are the resources relevant to the topic being studied? (yes or no)
   - Are the resources current? (yes or no)
   - How many resources given were published within the past 5 years? _____ the past 10 years? _____ or are older than 10 years? _____

10. **Ethical considerations**
    - Were ethical practices used when conducting the study? (yes or no)
    - If not, what was done in the study that you would consider unethical?

    _____

    _____

    _____

11. **Theoretical or conceptual framework**
    - Was a framework present or not? (yes or no) If so, can you identify it?

    _____

    _____

    _____

    - What type of theory or framework was used?

    _____

    _____

    _____

    - Was this theory or framework from the field of nursing? (yes or no)

12. **Operational terms**
    - Are operational terms given? (yes or no)
    - Are the terms appropriate for the given study? (yes or no)
    - Do they help clarify the study? (yes or no) Why or why not?

    _____

    _____

    _____

13. **Research design**
    - We have already classified the main type of research as quantitative or qualitative. Within that main classification,

what type of research is it (experimental or nonexperimental, phenomenological, etc.)?

_____

_____

_____

- What is the method used to assign subjects?

_____

_____

_____

- Was there randomization? (yes or no)
- Are there any variables? If so, list them below.

Variable 1:

_____

_____

_____

Variable 2:

_____

_____

_____

Variable 3:

_____

_____

_____

Variable 4:

_____

_____

_____

- Is any bias present? (yes or no) If so, list what you think is biased.

_____

_____

_____

- If the study has bias, think about why. Who funded the study? Who conducted the study? Where do the researchers work? Is a conflict of interest present?

_____

_____

_____

14. **Population and sample**
    - Who was studied?

    _____
    _____
    _____

    - What was the age group?

    _____
    _____
    _____

    - How many people were studied or used? What is the exact sample size?
      $n =$ _____
    - Do you think this is an adequate sample size? (yes or no) Why or why not?

    _____
    _____
    _____

15. What was the **data collection method** (survey, questionnaire, etc.) used?

    _____
    _____
    _____

16. Was the study **statistically significant?**
    - What are the p **values**?

    _____
    _____
    _____

    - What is the **confidence interval**?

    _____
    _____
    _____

17. Was this study significant to the field of nursing? (yes or no) Why or why not?

    _____
    _____
    _____

18. **Assumptions and limitations**
    - Did the author list any assumptions? (yes or no) If so, what were they?

    _____
    _____
    _____

- Did the author list any limitations? (yes or no) If so, what were they?

_____
_____
_____

19. What were the **conclusions?**

_____
_____
_____

20. **Implications for future research**
    - Were any implications or suggestions for future areas of research given by the author? (yes or no)
    - If so, what are they, and do you find them sensible and appropriate?

_____
_____
_____
_____
_____
_____
_____
_____
_____

REFERENCES

Carlson, D. S., Kruse, L. K., & Rouse, C. L. (1999). Critiquing nursing research. A user friendly guide for the staff nurse. *Journal of Emergency Nursing, 25*(4), 330–332. doi:10.1016/S0099-1767(99)70064-4

Fontana, R. J. (2008). Acute liver failure including acetaminophen overdose. *The Medical Clinics of North America, 92*(4), 761–794. doi:10.1016/j.mcna.2008.03.005

French, B. (2006). Evaluating research for use in practice: What criteria do specialist nurses use? *Journal of Advanced Nursing, 50*(3), 235–243. doi:10.1111/j.1365-2648.2005.03386.x

Long, C. O. (2009). Weighing in on the evidence. In N. Schmidt & J. Brown (Eds.), *Evidence based practice for nurses: Appraisal and application of research* (pp. 315–328). Boston, MA: Jones & Bartlett.

Malloch, K., & Porter-O'Grady, T. (2005). *Evidence-based practice in nursing and healthcare.* Sudbury, MA: Jones & Bartlett.

Melnyk, B. M., & Fineout-Overholt, E. (2010). *Evidence-based practice in nursing & healthcare: A guide to best practice* (2nd ed.). Philadelphia, PA: Lippincott Williams & Wilkins.

Newhouse, R. P., Dearholt, S., Poe, S., Pugh, L., & White, K. (2007). *Johns Hopkins nursing evidence-based practice: Model and guidelines.* Indianapolis, IN: Sigma Theta Tau International.

Sandelowski, M., & Barroso, J. (2002). Finding the findings in qualitative studies. *Journal of Nursing Scholarship, 34*(3), 213–219. doi:10.1111/j.1547-5069.2002.00213.x

United States Food and Drug Administration. (2018). *A guide to safe use of pain medicine.* Retrieved from https://www.fda.gov/ForConsumers/ConsumerUpdates/ucm095673.htm

9

Barriers to Disseminating the Evidence

This chapter examines some of the barriers to conducting research and implementing evidence-based practice (EBP) projects in nursing. Fear of the unknown and the effects of peer pressure, along with strong nursing traditions, sometimes inhibit the development of an EBP environment. In addition, organizational constraints, such as lack of administrative support or incentives to move forward with EBP, are explored. Finally, the chapter discusses how to overcome some of these obstacles.

In this chapter, you will learn:

1. The barriers to implementing EBP
2. How to change your practice environment
3. How technology affects EBP research
4. Ways to disseminate or present EBP research

BARRIERS TO SUCCESSFUL RESEARCH AND IMPLEMENTATION OF EBP

Chapter 1, Introduction to Evidence-Based Practice, mentioned various limitations to the implementation of EBP, including the following barriers to successful research:

- Lack of awareness or understanding of EBP
- Lack of association with researchers

- Lack of ability to locate or find relevant research
- Lack of ability to "understand the language" of research
- Lack of recognition of the value of research in nursing practice
- Lack of availability of computer databases
- Lack of basic knowledge of information technology
- Interpersonal issues (do not like writing, lack of confidence, lack of motivation, fear)
- Lack of time to obtain research information

These barriers are very real in the practice environment today. We must explore ways to eliminate them so that nursing can move forward as a profession. Patient-centered care requires that we practice nursing using the latest and best evidence to provide the best care possible for our patients. Collaboration with physicians and other healthcare practitioners is vital to building a collegial relationship based on trust, respect, and the best evidence. We must never tire of trying to find ways to implement EBP.

Australia and the United Kingdom have been leaders in the implementation of EBP. In the United States, EBP is increasingly being implemented in nursing. The move of hospital institutions to Magnet® status could be the impetus for this change. Recall from Chapter 1, Introduction to Evidence-Based Practice, that Magnet status is an award given by the American Nurses Credentialing Center (ANCC), an affiliate of the American Nurses Association, to hospitals that satisfy a set of criteria designed to measure the strength and quality of their nursing staffs. **A Magnet hospital is one in which nursing results in excellent patient outcomes, where nurses have a high level of job satisfaction, and where there is a low staff nurse turnover rate and appropriate grievance resolution.** Magnet status also indicates nurse involvement in data collection and decision making in patient care delivery. The idea behind this formal recognition is that Magnet nursing leaders value staff nurses, involve them in shaping research-based nursing practice, and encourage and reward them for advancing in nursing practice. Magnet hospitals are expected to have open communication between nurses and other members of the healthcare team and an appropriate personnel mix to attain the best patient outcomes and staff work environment (Center for Nursing Advocacy, 2007). This is accomplished by examining the current research trends and incorporating them into practice. Chapter 1 includes more information about this designation.

Fast Facts

A Magnet hospital is one in which nursing results in excellent patient outcomes, where nurses have a high level of job satisfaction, and where there is a low staff nurse turnover rate and appropriate grievance resolution.

But what do you do if the institution where you work is a smaller agency or does not have Magnet status? Where do you start to attract interest for EBP?

It is wise to first assess the particular barriers to EBP in your facility. You might accomplish this using a simple informal survey or a more formal focus group. A focus group brings together a small group of individuals to discuss a topic and respond to questions posed by a moderator or facilitator. For example, the topic could be the nursing staff's knowledge base, attitudes, beliefs, and thoughts regarding the research process and how to use research or evidence in practice. In addition, the focus group could be used to determine to what degree staff members believe implementing EBP will result in improved patient care or better outcomes. **If staff members do not believe that EBP will result in improved care and patient outcomes, the facilitator could provide examples or real-case scenarios of how this would occur.**

In addition, providing such examples, particularly those that produce cost savings, is well received by administrators and generally increases their willingness to consider implementing EBP. For example, if you work in a private nursing home and you are trying to implement an EBP environment, you might use the latest research to show that switching to an incontinence device that initially costs a dollar more than the device currently being used could eventually save hundreds of dollars in linen services and decubitus care, and this could result in better outcomes for patients. Presented in this way, the proposal is more likely to be taken under closer consideration by the administration. It is paramount for nurses to articulate the value of interventions within an economic framework that maintains institutional viability, and EBP provides a means to do so.

Fast Facts

If healthcare practitioners do not believe that EBP will result in improved care and patient outcomes, the facilitator needs to provide examples or real-case scenarios of how this would occur.

CHANGING THE PRACTICE ENVIRONMENT

Issues of nursing availability, productivity, working conditions, and the aging of the nursing workforce cannot be ignored. Today, many healthcare organizations are struggling to deal with the consequences of a decades-long nursing shortage. The move to restructure hospitals in the early 1990s resulted in reductions in the educated nursing workforce, ultimately threatening the clinical viability of these organizations at the same time that clinical interventions were becoming more complex. The productivity decisions made then have taken a large toll on the nursing resources of today's healthcare organizations. The historical lack of connection between the economic viability of these organizations and nursing satisfaction and performance is an important factor to consider when looking at the future financial and operational viability of healthcare organizations.

Nurses are indeed at the "crossroads of care" in the healthcare organization. It is the nurses' role to be the "eyes of the physician" and to quickly evaluate, coordinate, integrate, and facilitate all of the clinical functions related to the delivery of patient care. While this is a vital nursing function, nurses also must recognize the need to evaluate their clinical practice to determine whether it delivers optimal patient outcomes. This is where nursing must take the lead and be proactive. The process of reframing nursing calls for nurses to critically evaluate the clinical foundations of nursing practice as well as support healthcare institutions facing increased financial pressures. EBP is one method that nurses can use to improve patient outcomes. It takes the nurse from a previous focus only on the clinical process to a new focus that requires attention to clinical outcomes (Malloch & Porter-O'Grady, 2005).

Fast Facts

Nurses function at the "crossroads of care" in healthcare organizations. Their role is to be the "eyes of the physician" and to quickly evaluate, coordinate, integrate, and facilitate all of the clinical functions related to the delivery of patient care. But it is also vital that nurses evaluate the evidence associated with their clinical practice. EBP takes the nurse from a previous focus only on the clinical process to a new focus that requires attention to clinical outcomes.

TECHNOLOGY, DATABASES, AND EBP

It is imperative that the latest and best evidence be incorporated into EBP. This process is aided when nurses have access to the databases that contain information and research studies that can affect care. If your institution provides access to scientific databases, that is excellent. If it does not, obtain information about accessing the databases and the cost to acquire them, and then provide that information to the leaders or managers of your institution. As noted in Chapter 7, Finding the Evidence, some services, such as ScienceDirect, EBSCO, and OVID, provide databases for a fee and bundle packages for purchase. These services are an expensive proposition for smaller institutions, but an argument can be made that access to these databases will support the infrastructure of research and advancing science in your institution. **Make an argument for EBP.** You might also make an argument for a joint venture between departments or institutions to purchase the full-text online databases, thus decreasing the cost to an individual department or institution. "Buddying" with a local college or university that has a health sciences curriculum is another option. Remember that content for some journals included in these databases is not available electronically for up to a year. So, it may be wise to subscribe to important research journals or encourage staff to go directly to journal websites that offer free access to their most recent issues, as well as **e-zines** and **e-journals** that are available on the Internet (see Chapter 7, Finding the Evidence).

LACK OF KNOWLEDGE ABOUT EBP

It is vital that classes be offered to educate the staff about EBP. Lack of knowledge about EBP or fear of the unknown is sometimes the single most important barrier to convincing colleagues to get on board and understand the process. In a 2002 study, Jolly noted that nurses' attitudes toward research and development were poor until a program was developed to assist them in understanding how to read and critically appraise research articles. Programs or classes may be held as formal or informal inservice education to assist in this process.

Many nurses are fearful not only about the process of searching for research articles but also about what to do with them when they find them. Addressing this knowledge gap should be a focus of future educational development. As more nurses are required to take research courses, the question must be asked: Do those courses go far enough in deciphering for enrollees what to do with the research studies they find to change practice? This text was written with the goal of providing a guide to simplify this often daunting and overwhelming task and alleviate the bedside nurse's fear of the EBP process.

Along with providing your support, which is invaluable in alleviating fears, encourage your peers to visit databases, such as the Cochrane Library and the National Guidelines Clearinghouse (discussed in Chapter 1, Introduction to Evidence-Based Practice), which provide completed systematic reviews and EBP guidelines for implementation. Check local colleges and universities for courses about EBP. Online resources for learning about EBP are also available through nursing schools, and selected centers have developed around the world with the primary purpose of promoting EBP (see Table 9.1). Even when nurses understand research, many do not have the skills to access evidence or evaluate it for potential decision making (Polit & Beck, 2016).

Table 9.1

Online Resources for Tutorials on Evidence-Based Practice

Online Resource	Website
AANA (American Association of Nurse Anesthetists), free EBP tutorial	https://www.aana.com/practice/evidence-based-practice
Center for Advancing Clinical Excellence at the University of Texas Health Science Center at San Antonio	http://nursing.uthscsa.edu/onrs/starmodel/
Center for Health Evidence	http://www.cche.net/
Center for Research and Evidence-Based Practice at the University of Rochester School of Nursing	https://son.rochester.edu/research/center-research-support.html
Joanna Briggs Institute	www.joannabriggs.org
Sara Cole Hirsh Institute for Best Nursing Practice Based on Evidence at the Frances Payne Bolton School of Nursing, Case Western Reserve University	fpb.case.edu/Centers/Hirsh

Melnyk and Fineout-Overholt (2010) analyzed 44 systematic reviews focusing on the effects of strategies to change the practice of healthcare professionals. They noted that little research had been done to develop and sustain EBP and drew the following conclusions:

- Passive dissemination of research is ineffective.
- A range of interventions has been shown to be effective in changing the behavior of healthcare professionals.
- Multifaceted interventions are more likely to be effective than a single intervention.
- Individual practitioners' beliefs, attitudes, and knowledge influence their behavior, but other factors, including organizational, economic, and community environments, also are important.
- A diagnostic analysis should be conducted to identify barriers and supportive factors likely to influence the proposed change in practice.
- Successful strategies to change practice need to be adequately resourced and require people with appropriate knowledge and skills.

The diverse personalities, health professionals, and clinical settings that make up today's healthcare organizations underscore the importance of involving more resources and support as well as effecting a paradigm and culture shift in the organization. Strategies suggested by Melnyk and Fineout-Overholt (2010) include:

- One-on-one sessions between health professional educators and individual staff to explain the desired practice change or the concepts of EBP
- Print and computerized reminders to prompt the practitioner's behavior change in practice
- Educational meetings or inservice education that requires active participation of the learners
- Audits and feedback in which clinical performance is monitored through electronic database or chart review
- Direct observation and feedback

Other sources suggest these additional strategies:

- Involvement of unit-based committees, such as performance improvement (PI), quality assurance (QA), or policy and procedure committee members, to facilitate the EBP process.
- Journal or research article clubs that enhance the discussion of a particular article per month. Several studies (Jolly, 2002; Karkos &

Peters, 2006; McQueen, Miller, Nivison, & Husband, 2006) found that journal clubs increased awareness, knowledge, confidence, and skills in research.

- Poster presentations in which units within an institution share with the entire healthcare institution ideas and EBP projects created, ongoing, or developed by each unit.
- A nursing research day, with presentations and seminars to encourage participation and facilitate understanding of EBP.

OFFERING INCENTIVES

Incentives are a motivational tool that can be used to stimulate interest and bring about change in the workplace environment. Contests can be arranged, with prizes given. Providing free food is one way to improve attendance at an EBP program. Free T-shirts, book bags, or pens are other ways of generating interest and increasing attendance. A simple gift of a chocolate bar for attendance might suffice as a motivational factor for some. Survey the population you will be working with, and provide incentives of interest to that group.

INCLUDING EBP IN PERFORMANCE APPRAISALS

Another idea that managers can use to implement and facilitate environmental change is to require involvement in EBP as part of annual performance appraisals. A monetary incentive tied to employees' annual appraisals can be a great motivating force to move staff toward involvement in the EBP process. When you make EBP part of your "unit culture," it will become a real process that is valued by the administration. You can make a difference, particularly in providing great patient care and cost savings, for the institution in which you work.

TIME AND SUPPORT

Most important, administrators must realize that they cannot expect nurses to "fit" research and EBP into their normal daily care schedule. Most managers recognize the rigor and demands of the clinical work environment, and that time away from the job must be allotted to encourage participation and interest. Administrative support for this process is vital. It is well worth the time involved to present the EBP process to management and enlist the support of the administration before embarking on the EBP process. Staff release time or paid conference time is vital, as is encouraging your institution to facilitate research by buying into research databases, or "buddying" or sharing the cost with a local college or university. In this way, healthcare professionals support EBP and each other.

DISSEMINATING THE EVIDENCE

Once you have gained interest and support for EBP, new and exciting projects can be planned and implemented. Do not forget to share your results with colleagues. So much of the wonderful work done in nursing is never published or shared. The following are a few ways through which we can share our efforts and successes in moving the science of nursing forward.

PRESENTING EBP INFORMATION

EBP projects and successful implementation strategies can be presented at local conferences, national conferences, or intrahospital inservice educational programs. Publication in a nursing journal is a way of reaching a larger audience to disseminate important work.

Oral Presentations

When presenting the information you have developed about an EBP project, be both systematic and organized. Most conference presentations are approximately 20 to 30 minutes long. A good rule is to allow 1 minute per PowerPoint slide (if using PowerPoint). Allow time for questions. When planning a presentation, be clear and concise. If presenting PowerPoint slides, be sure the type size used on the slides is at least 24 point in the selected font so that attendees can read them clearly from the back of the room. Titles should be slightly larger, and references can be 16 point.

You should also use sharp and contrasting colors that are easily read in a large room. Use black when writing on a white background and white when writing on a black background. Avoid the overuse of clip art or pictures that will detract from your professional presentation.

Tips:

- Do not overdo the content. New presenters tend to try to cover too much. Identify key pieces of information, and do not overload the audience.

- Vary slide graphics and layout but not so much that it is distracting. Avoid overuse of extreme colors.
- Use titles on the slides to help audience understand content.
- Use graphs when possible. They are easier to read than tables.
- Author names and a date should be included for direct citations or a specific research study. Place these citations directly on the slide in a smaller font. Complete references should be cited at the end and available for attendees.
- Proofread and check spelling multiple times.
- Save your presentation. Back it up in multiple places. Submit it in accordance with conference specifications, but always take a backup copy on a flash drive or on your own computer. Email your presentation to yourself if the file is not too large.
- Try to engage the audience through eye contact or active participation versus lecturing to the attendees. Ask questions to the audience to engage them.
- Allow time for questions and clarifications.
- Be available after the presentation to clarify and network with conference attendees.
- Have business cards available with your email to hand out.

To organize your content, start by making an outline. **Start every presentation with objectives or a list of the outcomes you want the learner to achieve.** Then clearly present your EBP project. You can use the following steps:

1. Introduce your clinical problem or EBP topic.
2. State the purpose you hoped to achieve with your project or problem of interest. What is it that you wanted to change in practice, or what inspired you to examine this topic?
3. Include any theoretical or conceptual frameworks that may have guided your work (not usually used in EBP but more often included in a nursing research project).
4. Detail the interventions you implemented or examined in your EBP project.
5. **Provide a brief summary of the evidence.** This can be done in a table using the format and style recommended by the American Psychological Association (APA). (See Chapter 11, Examples of a PICOT Process, for examples of evidence tables.) You may want to include the ranking or hierarchy of evidence (e.g., randomized controlled trial [RCT], level 1, or highest and strongest type of evidence). You may also want to include clinical practice guidelines that have already been established.
6. What did you find in conducting your project that led (or did not lead) to a practice change? This is a summary of your findings.

Conclude with implications that your findings will have for future practice, and mention areas where additional research may be needed.

This presentation can take place live in a conference, an institutional, or a clinical setting, or as a poster presentation. More information about these methods follows.

Panel Discussions

Panel discussions are sometimes used to share and discuss the findings of EBP issues or research. The panel is usually a group of experts in the field but could be a group of students or nurses who completed an EBP project. Before the discussion, determine the allotted amount of time for each speaker and which speaker will handle which topic. Find out how the panel will be moderated and by whom. Remember to allow a question-and-answer period to encourage the audience to participate in the discussion. This can be done in a professional conference setting or informally in an institutional or a clinical setting.

Poster Presentations

Poster presentations are probably the easiest way to disseminate current nursing information. Poster presentations may be given at local or national conferences. Sharing information at a national conference provides important and timely information for colleagues and practitioners. The methods of composing and sharing the poster differ depending on the type of organization sponsoring the event. Be sure to check the requirements for submitting an abstract of a poster, and the actual poster criteria, before sending any information. Many conferences have size requirements and may or may not provide instruments to hang the poster if needed. The typical size for a poster is 4 feet by 6 feet. It is also important to plan the graphics and pictures incorporated in a poster. The golden rule is for the attendee at the conference to be able to view the poster from 4 feet away. Some other items to consider in presenting a poster are as follows:

- Consider the audience attending the conference, including the language of the attendees. Do the members speak primarily English? Are they professional medical people or laypeople? For laypeople, medical jargon may be confusing.
- Make the poster readable. Vary the size of the font used in the poster. Do not make the letters too small or too large, or they will detract from the content of the poster. The conference attendee should be able to read the poster highlights from 4 feet away.

- Use pictures or graphics only when they add to the content of your poster. A few graphics are eye pleasing if they are relevant, but too many graphics make the poster look "busy" and can frustrate the reader.
- Use a font that is easy to read. Consider the typical fonts you use to write a paper, such as Times New Roman or Arial. Use the same font throughout the poster. You can use a special or decorative font, such as comic sans, at a pediatric conference if it is appropriate for the type of conference.
- Avoid shadowing the letters. This can make them hard to read.
  - Consider outsourcing the poster to an outside company. It may save you money. All you need to do is put your information in PowerPoint format and send via email. Check with the individual vendor for requirements especially if incorporating photos (may need jpeg file).
- Consider providing attendees with handouts that summarize your poster, and provide your contact information. You may also want to provide a list of references. You can also distribute business cards that attendees can take to their own practice environment and share with their colleagues. These handouts can be in color or black and white. The handouts can be an outline of your information or a copy of the poster itself. Consider cost when making handouts. Color is obviously more expensive.
- Be present at your poster during scheduled poster exhibit times to answer any questions that conference attendees may have. This also gives you time to network with other professionals in your practice area.
  - Do not forget pushpins. They are not always provided. You do not want to get to a conference and then have no way to hang your poster.
  - Do consider how you will transport the poster to the conference especially if traveling by plane. It may be easier just to mail it there. Pick it up on arrival at the conference mail center.

Small Group Presentations

The results of your EBP study can be shared in small groups at a multitude of places. This can be done among a few (three to six) of your peers or colleagues over a lunch or dinner break; on the clinical unit or in a classroom or auditorium; through a grand rounds–type presentation; through professional committee meetings (either unit based or hospital- or institution-wide); or, if relevant, in the community or at a comparable agency or worksite.

Professional Publications

Did you ever wonder who writes the articles in the journals you read? The answer is people just like you. If you develop an EBP project or simply want to share the review of literature you compiled, **consider publishing your findings in a professional journal** or publication. Remember journals can be published in a print version or online in an electronic version. There are a wide range of publication options, which include nursing specialty journals, medical and other healthcare journals, websites, electronic journals, and web publications. Important today are blogs and podcasts as well, but not usually for publication.

Many nurses are apprehensive about the process of submitting an article for publication and uncertain how to do so. However, the process is usually quite easy and not something to fear. The following suggestions can help as you begin this process:

1. *First, identify an idea or topic of interest.* What types of nursing are you interested in? What field of nursing is your interest or expertise? What is your passion? What happens in your clinical work area that bothers you or piques your curiosity so that you want to learn more about it? Identify an issue. You can consult your peers, do some brainstorming, or look in the journals you receive. Many times there are sections or a page in the journal citing areas of interest in publishing, such as EBP topics, ethical issues, practice issues, and new procedures or products.
2. *Write your article*, or conduct your EBP project. If you need assistance, consider a mentor. Speak with a colleague or an associate who has published. Consult a previous instructor or professor.
3. *Proofread* or have others read and critique your work. Asking for insight and suggestions to improve your work may sometimes create the tone and excitement for EBP.
4. *Select a journal of interest related to your topic.* It certainly would not be appropriate to write an article or EBP project focused on a pediatric issue such as immunizations and then seek to publish it in a geriatric or an emergency/trauma journal. Select a journal that is relevant to the topic of interest.
5. *Follow the journal's guidelines for submission*, which are usually posted online on its website and can also be found on the masthead of print editions. Steps 4 and 5 are discussed in more detail below.

In most cases you will want to select a journal that is scholarly or peer reviewed. **A peer-reviewed journal is one that is reviewed**

by a panel of experts in the field. Peer-reviewed journals are more intensely reviewed than those reviewed by another process. This is the ideal and most respected type of publication. However, if this is your first submission, you may want to submit your work to a non-peer-reviewed journal. Again, follow the guidelines for that type of journal. There is nothing wrong with "trying the process out" with this type of journal. As you progress in your scholarly work, it is best, however, that you publish in peer-reviewed journals.

As mentioned, the requirements for submission of a manuscript can be found either in the journal or on its website. To locate a journal's guidelines online, enter the name of the journal into your search engine, go to the journal's home page, and then look for "guidelines for authors" or "author submissions." Follow them exactly to avoid time-wasting delays or rejection of your submission. The journal may recommend that you submit a **letter of query**. This is simply a letter sent to the editors, telling them that you have written a manuscript about a particular topic and asking if the editorial board would be interested in looking at it. If you receive a positive response, you would then submit the manuscript. If the response is negative, you should look for another journal until you find one that is interested in your subject area or topic of interest.

Information covered in the author submission guidelines includes:

- The length of the manuscript
- The type of paper and size on which it is to be submitted
- The required font and its size
- Spacing requirements
- Requirements for abstracts
- Style for bibliographies; for nursing journals, this is usually APA format
- How to organize the body of the manuscript
- How to handle graphics, tables, or charts
- A description of the review process and the timeline for feedback to the author

These items vary by publication, and there may be different sets of guidelines depending on whether you are submitting your manuscript electronically or as a hard copy (typed format). Most manuscripts are now submitted electronically. Some journals also use submission software that allows the author to establish an account and check the status of the manuscript online at the publisher's website. Just remember to follow the author guidelines closely. Swanson, McCloskey, and Bodensteiner (1991) surveyed 92 nursing journals to determine the main reason for manuscript rejection. The highest ranked reason was that they were poorly written. This was also cited in a survey by McConnell (2000). Other reasons for manuscript rejection cited by Swanson et al. (1991) were undocumented content, unimportant content, clinically inapplicable findings, statistical problems, incorrectly interpreted data, and overly technical content.

Mee (2003) shares the following nine lessons on writing for publication, which are still relevant for today:

1. *Be confident.* You can be a nurse author. Writing is not just for those in academic settings. Many nurses like to read about other nurses in similar situations and how they solved problems.
2. *Start small.* Do not overwhelm yourself with a large topic such as pneumonia. Find an aspect of the broader topic you are passionate about, and explore it.
3. *Topic development takes time and effort.* Many nurses are intimidated and think ideas just pop into a writer's head. The truth is that many authors take a lot of time to develop their topic and focus.
4. *Gather more resources than you think you will need.* Conduct a literature search, and then read all the articles you have found. Immerse yourself in the topic. Writing will be easier if you know the topic well.
5. *Know the journal you want to write for.* There are more than 150 nursing journals, both general and specialized. Choose 3 journals that you think might be a good fit for your article. Then read those journals to see if the articles match your style. Follow the author guidelines, and do not forget to submit a letter of interest or a query letter.
6. *Start writing in the middle.* Do not waste time trying to come up with the perfect title. Get the ideas on paper as a rough draft, and then go back to fix and clarify your points. Just start writing.
7. *Use the active rather than the passive voice.* The active voice connects with the reader. In contrast, the passive voice is indirect, vague, and puts distance between the author and the reader.
8. Multiple rewrites are the norm, so *plan for at least three rewrites.*
9. Lastly, *pay attention to detail.* Again follow the author guidelines, and put together a cleanly written and organized manuscript. Careless errors in spelling or punctuation will undermine your credibility as a writer with the editor. Then walk away and wait. Once this process is completed and you see your name in print as an author, you will have a sense of pride and accomplishment like you have never known. So, go for it, take a chance, and write (Mee, 2003).

Fast Facts

Remember that the process of publishing an article in a professional journal can be a long one. An article often will not be published for several months, and the lag time to publication may approach a year. This diminishes the timeliness of important research. The best way to transmit current research information to your peers in a timely fashion is to present it at a conference. Whichever method you choose, make sure that you do share your research. This is how the body of nursing knowledge will grow—if we all share and collaborate.

REFERENCES

Center for Nursing Advocacy. (2016). *Magnet status: What it is, what it is not, and what it could be.* Retrieved from http://www.nursingadvocacy.org/faq/magnet.html

Jolly, S. (2002). Raising research awareness: A strategy for nurses. *Nursing Standard, 16*(33), 33–39. doi:10.7748/ns2002.05.16.33.33.c3188

Karkos, B., & Peters, K. A. (2006). A magnet community hospital: Fewer barriers to nursing research utilization. *Journal of Nursing Administration, 36*(7), 377–382. Retrieved from https://journals.lww.com/jonajournal/Abstract/2006/07000/A_Magnet_Community_Hospital__Fewer_Barriers_to.11.aspx

Malloch, K., & Porter-O'Grady, T. (2005). *Evidence-based practice in nursing and healthcare.* Sudbury, MA: Jones & Bartlett.

McConnell, E. A. (2000). Nursing publications outside the United States. *Journal of Nursing Scholarship, 32*, 87–92. doi:10.1111/j.1547-5069.2000.00087.x

McQueen, J., Miller, C., Nivison, C., & Husband, V. (2006). An investigation into the use of a journal club for evidence based practice. *International Journal of Therapy and Rehabilitation, 13*(7), 311–316. doi:10.12968/ijtr.2006.13.7.21407

Mee, C. L. (2003). Ten lessons in writing for publication. *Journal of Infusion Nursing, 26*(2), 110–113. doi:10.1097/00129804-200303000-00008

Melnyk, B. M., & Fineout-Overholt, E. (2010). *Evidence-based practice in nursing & healthcare: A guide to best practice* (2nd ed.). Philadelphia, PA: Lippincott Williams & Wilkins.

Polit, D. G., & Beck, C. T. (2016). *Nursing research: Generating and assessing evidence for nursing practice* (10th ed.). Philadelphia, PA: Wolters Kluwer.

Swanson, E. A., McCloskey, J. C., & Bodensteiner, A. (1991). Publishing opportunities for nurses: A comparison of 92 U.S. journals. *Image: Journal of Nursing Scholarship, 23*, 33–38. doi:10.1111/j.1547-5069.1991.tb00632.x

10

Evidence-Based Practice in the Nurse Residency Program

Upon graduating nursing school and entering into practice, many nurses enroll in nurse residency programs (NRPs) in hospitals, particularly those accredited by The Joint Commission. Part of such programs is the completion of an evidence-based practice (EBP) project by the new graduate nurse. This chapter is presented as a guide to help you understand and develop an EBP project.

In this chapter you will learn:

1. To understand the NRPs
2. Steps to develop an EBP project and come up with an idea
3. How to form a team
4. Ways to grade the evidence
5. How to implement practice change
6. Ways to disseminate and share your work

INTRODUCTION TO NRPs

Nursing seems to be challenged by recurring workplace shortages. One of the issues is the excessive loss of newly licensed registered nurses (NLRNs). Almost one in five leaves during the 1st year of practice. One in three will leave within the first 2 years (Kovner,

Nurse residency programs were developed to help new graduate nurses transition into clinical practice. These programs typically last about 6 to 12 months.

The Institute of Medicine (2010) report recommends that every nurse should have the benefit of having a nurse residency program at the beginning of their career and whenever making a transition in their career.

Brewer, Fatehi, & Jun, 2014). The cost of orienting new registered nurses (RNs) only to have to replace them has forced institutions to look at ways to enhance retention. Sometimes what is missed is socialization into the role of nursing. Kramer (1974) mentioned this as "reality shock" that was experienced as new graduates transition from the role of student nurse to newly graduated nurse and suggests that the lack of socialization is why they left nursing. Evidence supports the use of transitioning programs to retain new graduates. One of these transition-to-practice programs is the NRP. Many hospitals and institutions have tried to combat this issue of high turnover by developing an NRP. Part of the NRP is to develop an EBP project during the time of the residency. Also important to note is that the Institute of Medicine (IOM), National Council of the State Board of Nursing (NCSBN), Quality and Safety Education for Nurses (QSEN) initiative, and Magnet® facilities all recommend infusing EBP competencies into NRPs. Adequate time needs to be given for NRPs. In a study by Jackson (2016), evidence was found to support the need to extend nursing residencies beyond 6 months and/or to individualize EBP training within NRPs. Also found was the need for further research on the appropriate timing of EBP training during NRPs as well as determining the readiness of new graduates for EBP training (Warren, Perkins, & Greene, 2016).

Some companies have developed curricula for NRPs. One of them is Vizient. While we are not endorsing this company or product, just know that the NRP of Vizient/American Association of Colleges of Nursing (AACN) is one of the first of its kind to help transition NLRNs into their clinical roles and build confidence. They have developed an EBP curriculum and final project. They also provide interactive exercises. The goal was to decrease turnover rate, improve decision making, enhance leadership, and implement EBP into practice. Many hospital systems are using this program. It guides the NLRN through developing an EBP project, which at the end, they can present to the unit or at a conference as posters or presentations. A booklet is provided for NLRNs to work through the steps of developing an EBP project. It can be tailored to meet the needs of an individual hospital or institution. The focus of this chapter is to discuss how to facilitate an EBP project not only for NRPs or internships but for all new graduate nurses.

Fast Facts

Nurse residency programs extend beyond traditional orientation programs to engage and empower new nurses to be critical thinkers and leaders at the bedside.

STARTING THE PROCESS

During orientation to the NRP, new RNs will be given clinical schedules and requirements. Many will be told that part of their residency is the development of an EBP project. Most have the entire time of their residency (varies from 6 months to a year) to complete this project. This project is usually done in groups. Working in smaller groups may make it easier to work out schedules and find time to meet and discuss. Smaller groups can allow for more involvement with the research process and ownership when it is completed. Perhaps the hardest part of the project is to come up with an EBP idea. This is hard to do when new to a unit. Know that as orientation starts the RN begins to observe, wonder, and ask why. Why do you do that procedure like that? Why is this done that way? Is this practice decision based on research? Is this a clinical practice guideline? Does it work? If not, should it be changed? These are some of the observations a new RN should be able to make. That being said, some are so overwhelmed they do not have time or the critical thinking skills or experience to choose a topic. So this process may take a few months to come up with an idea. The clinical nurse educator (CNE) or specialist of the unit is usually the organizer or driving force with this process. It may be followed up and final approval given for a project by the division of education (DOE). But how do you pick a topic or idea?

Ways to Decide on an EBP Idea

The following are some categories of EBP ideas for consideration. The idea can look at nurses themselves and how they function and cope. The idea could be unit procedure or practice based or driven by administration to remain in compliance with regulatory agencies. The idea could flow from one unit into another as well as enhance communication between colleagues and/or departments within the institution. Table 10.1 shows the general ideas and questions to ask in order to come up with a specific idea for an EBP project. In no way is the list exhaustive or complete; it's just a basis for brainstorming to get you thinking.

Do any of these ideas strike an interest or make you think of something that may be appropriate for your unit/floor? If so, great. If not, while on orientation, just keep asking yourself, "Why do we do it this way? Does it make sense?" Ask that very question to other staff members, and if they say "I don't know. That is just how we always did it," that should be a red flag to investigate further into the process. If you are still stuck, ask the unit nurses who have been working there. They will usually be able to come up with a minimum of 10 ideas to get you started that they themselves have wondered about or seen as problematic. The unit staff are your best resource. You could also ask your unit educator. Through compliance monitoring, unit education, and personal experience, they know the flow of the unit best and can lead you down the right path. They can also help you narrow a broad topic or expand on a topic that is too selective. They need to be your partner and facilitator of this process. Lastly, whatever you choose for a specific topic, make sure you are interested in it or passionate about it. Just like someone doing a research project, if you do not have passion for your topic, you will lose interest in it. You will need to find evidence and research on it, so you want to like the topic. Do not let one be assigned to you by an educator or leadership team (sometimes this may happen depending on the needs of the unit). While it may be needed for your particular unit, if you have no interest in the topic, this process will be less rewarding for you. Once you have found a topic of interest to you, you need to sell it to others to get them excited about it too! One word of caution: If you are planning to select a topic that could cause a major clinical practice change, be sure to get buy-in from administration and physician staff *prior* to starting your project, or it will be a waste of time. How do you know for sure? Ask your unit-specific clinical educator. Another important thing to consider is to make yourself a timeline for doing things and try to stick to it. This process takes time, and if you are given 6 months to accomplish it, you do not want to wait until the last few weeks and rush the process.

Table 10.1

Ideas and Questions to Ask to Come Up With a Specific Idea for an EBP Project

Idea	Questions to Ask Yourself/Topics to Consider
Personal/nurse survival	How do new nurses survive the 1st year? What does being competent mean? Respect between team and unit ■ RN–RN ■ RN–MD ■ RN–Leadership/management PTSD in nursing Compassion fatigue Moral distress Burnout
Unit procedures/protocols/practices	■ Why do we do it this way? ■ Can we do it better? ■ Transfer criteria to lower level (Is it still safe?) ■ Transfer of patients ■ Admission of patients ■ Rounding on the floor/unit (Is nursing included?) ■ Patient care issues (Is nursing included and does it have input into the decision-making of the unit flow or practice environment?) ■ What are the procedures you spend a lot of time doing or do frequently? ■ Is there a new practice in the organization (e.g., policy) that needs to be implemented? ■ Do you know of a new protocol (i.e., policy, procedure, or standard) that could improve practice?
Disease or illness driven	This list can be limitless depending on the unit in which you work: ■ Patency of central lines ■ Use of alteplase (tPA), by who? ■ Policy/procedure ■ How we take temperatures ■ Ventilator/oxygen weaning ■ **Medication errors** ■ Why does the lab lose specimens, and why do I need to recollect? ■ Where could cost savings be achieved?
Patient or family/caregiver driven	■ What questions are patients and families asking? ■ What issues are patients/families identifying in person or on surveys as problematic or in need of a process change? ■ Who are the high-volume patients? ■ Who are the patients with the highest risk for a poor outcome? ■ Where is care missing in daily practice (cultural or comfort interventions)?

(continued)

Table 10.1

Ideas and Questions to Ask to Come Up With a Specific Idea for an EBP Project (*continued*)

Idea	Questions to Ask Yourself/Topics to Consider
	■ What common patient/family experiences could be improved?
	■ Has patient/family shared their experience in a way you had not anticipated?
Safety	Is this safe practice?
	Falls
	Review The Joint Commission's National Patient Safety Goals:
	■ Identify patients correctly using name and date of birth
	■ Improve staff communication
	■ Use medicines safely
	■ Use alarms safely
	■ Prevent infections
	■ Identify patient safety risks
	■ Prevent mistakes in surgery
	Is the environment where I work safe? Can I make it safer?
	Are there safety screening tools, and do they work?
	What one thing could I change to make this unit safer for patients, families, and staff?
	Are the sleep practices safe? Do they work? Are we practicing them consistently?
	Lateral violence in healthcare
Communication	Shift-to-shift report (Is it effective and working? Bedside report vs. at the desk)
	Communication with physicians
	Communication between departments
	Use of the phone: Can I get a direct number versus going through a phone loop inside the hospital?
	Is my patient/family communicating well with the physicians? Are their questions being answered?
Compliance with regulating agencies	Look at the AACN's healthy work standards. Do we have these, or how can we make these better?
	■ Skilled communication (SBAR and intercollaborative)
	■ True collaboration of all team players
	■ Effective decision making
	■ Appropriate staffing
	■ Meaningful recognition
	■ Authentic leadership
	What are National Patient Safety Goals for improving quality care?
	Documentation
Ethical issues	End-of-life-care practices
	Declaring brain death
	Organ donation

(continued)

Table 10.1

Ideas and Questions to Ask to Come Up With a Specific Idea for an EBP Project (*continued*)

Idea	Questions to Ask Yourself/Topics to Consider
	Futile care Palliative care The family who cannot let go
Physical issues	Layout: Is this unit designed right? Do my feet hurt at the end of the day? Why? Is this room design functional? Can I see the monitor? Do we have the right equipment? Can I access it easily? Does it work as it was designed?

AACN, American Association of Colleges of Nursing; PTSD, posttraumatic stress disorder; SBAR, situation, background, assessment, recommendation.

Form Your Team

Once you have your topic chosen, then you will need to form your team. In NRPs you will work with anywhere from one other nurse or partner to a group of five or six. Be sure all on your team are as interested in the topic as you are. If the entire group is not on board, the workload may not be evenly distributed, and the project may founder. Choose a team leader who reaches out to check in on everyone and keeps the group moving forward. Find a champion (usually the clinical educator) to help you move your initiative forward. You may also want to include a physician on the team depending on the topic. This physician serve as a resource, guide, or consultant with limited input when needed. Remember team members who are not RNs might only be on your team for a brief period of time. For example, if you need help collecting data, you might want to employ an IT (information technology) person. That person can assist you in gathering data, but does not need to remain on the team until completion, just for a portion of the process.

Find, Grade, and Critique the Evidence

Some find this part the second hardest, after coming up with a topic idea. Do not be overwhelmed. Consult a librarian if you have difficulty finding the evidence. See Chapter 7, Finding the Evidence. Look for existing EBP guidelines, clinical pathways, or research. There are several methods available for grading the evidence.

The easiest way would be to assign a simple A, B, and C: A = scientific evidence provided by well-conducted controlled trials (randomized or nonrandomized) with statistically significant results that support the recommendation; B = scientific evidence provided by observational studies or by controlled trials with less consistent results; and C = expert opinion. You can use expert opinion if scientifically consistent results were not present or available or if controlled trials were lacking (LoBiondo-Wood & Haber, 2014). A very easy guide to understanding the level of importance of research is to look at the "Schematic of Evidence Hierarchy" pyramid (see Figure 8.1 in Chapter 8, Evaluating the Evidence). This was developed by Polit and Beck (2016). There is also a rating system for the hierarchy of evidence (from Melnyk & Fineout-Overholt, 2010). See Box 1.2 in Chapter 1, Introduction to Evidence-Based Practice.

Another part is critiquing the evidence you have found. There are many ways to do that. Critical areas that should be considered when evaluating evidence are as follows: date of publication (you want the newest evidence possible, obviously not old evidence or research, preferably within the last 5 years), who wrote it, was it endorsed by anyone, did it have a clear purpose for whom it was designed, what types of evidence was it (research or nonresearch), and was it tested or implemented in practice? There are tables in this book to assist you in critiquing quantitative research (Table 5.2 in Chapter 5, Quantitative Research) and in critiquing qualitative research (Table 6.2 in Chapter 6, Qualitative Research). This will help you decide if there is enough evidence to guide and potentially change clinical practice.

PUTTING FORTH EBP RECOMMENDATIONS

Based on the critique of current EBP guidelines and the literature, make recommendations for practice change. Consult team members and your point person (who may be the unit-based educator), and put in writing your recommendations for practice change based on the evidence you found. Remember practice should NEVER be changed based on only one article or research study. That is not enough evidence.

Decision to Change Clinical Practice

Once the studies are critiqued and nicely synthesized into an evidence document, the next step is to decide, along with the team, if it is appropriate to put forth to change clinical practice. Things you might want to consider:

Is the evidence relevant for practice?

Was there consistency in findings across studies and EBP guidelines (if any)?

Feasibility for use in clinical practice: Will it work?

What is the risk–benefit ratio? Will it cause harm to patients or be of benefit to them?

It is recommended that the practice change be implemented *only* if it is based on knowledge/evidence derived from several sources (quality research studies) that demonstrate *consistent* findings (LoBiondo-Wood & Haber, 2014).

Finalize Your Development of EBP

Put your plan in writing using a consistent grading scheme that has been agreed upon. A written EBP standard and policies and procedures or guidelines need to be developed and written. They should then become part of the institution's policy and procedure manual. Most policies and procedures need to be reviewed by multiple nurses and administrators. They may need to be approved by your institution's nursing practice counsel, division of education department, and/or administration.

Implementing the Change

Consider doing this in a step-by-step or phased manner. You might want to start out with a pilot or trial implementation phase and then integrate it into practice. What is important to remember is that in order to implement change, you need to lock into the social system in the place you work. The role of the nurse manager is critical in making EBP changes at the bedside. Advance practice nurses (APNs) are helpful in retrieving and critiquing the studies and other evidence on a given topic (LoBiondo-Wood & Haber, 2016).

What to Do If Change Is Not Indicated

What happens if, after completing your EBP, your results are not as you anticipated? What do you do then? Do you rework your PICOT questions? Do you suggest further research to find out why the expected outcome was not reached? What if you find out that current practice in your institution is correct and should not be changed? Do not give up on a project just because the outcome did not meet your expectations. Try to figure out why you got the outcome you did. There could be many reasons. Regroup, have a debriefing, and discuss your findings. Employ someone with more research experience to assist you. Do not give up! Get support. Your unit educator can guide you and offer some suggestions. Do know that you personally are not a failure because your project did not yield your anticipated results.

Disseminate and Share Your Work

A significant part of this project is that you will learn collaboration in working with your peers and colleagues. As a new RN, this will give you a great opportunity to network with other employees/departments/individuals that gives you a sense of "community" in the workplace so you do not feel so "alone." EBPs may be a way for the NLRN to take pride and ownership in the new workplace, thus increasing the retention rate. Part of this process is sharing what you have done via a poster, podium presentation, or publication.

REFERENCES

Institute of Medicine. (2010). *The future of nursing: Leading change, advancing health*. Washington, DC: National Academies Press.

Jackson, J. (2016). Incorporating evidence-based practice learning into a nurse residency program: Are new graduates ready to apply evidence at the bedside? *Journal of Nursing Administration, 46*(5), 278–283. doi:10.1097/NNA.0000000000000343

Kovner, C. T., Brewer, C. S., Fatehi, F., & Jun, J. (2014). What does nurse turnover rate mean and what is the rate? *Policy, Politics, & Nursing Practice, 15*(3–4), 64–71. doi:10.1177/1527154414547953

Kramer, M. (1974). *Reality shock; why nurses leave nursing*. St. Louis, MO: C. V. Mosby.

LoBiondo-Wood, G., & Haber, J. (2014). *Nursing research: Methods and critical appraisal for evidence based practice* (8th ed.). St. Louis, MO: C. V. Mosby.

Melnyk, B. M., & Fineout-Overholt, E. (2010). *Evidence-based practice in nursing & healthcare: A guide to best practice* (2nd ed.). Philadelphia, PA: Lippincott Williams & Wilkins.

Polit, D. G., & Beck, C. T. (2016). *Nursing research: Generating and assessing evidence for nursing practice* (10th ed.). Philadelphia, PA: Wolters Kluwer.

Warren, J., Perkins, S., & Greene, M. A. (2016). Advancing new nurse graduate education through implementation of statewide, standardized nurse residency programs. *Journal of Nursing Regulation, 8*(4), 14–21. doi:10.1016/S2155-8256(17)30177-1

11

Examples of a PICOT Process

EXAMPLE 1

Step 1: Come Up With the Idea

EBP Project: Placement of postpyloric feeding tubes in the pediatric ICU (PICU)

The interest in this topic evolved from working with the pediatric population in the PICU and observing the decreased incidence of aspiration pneumonia. The occurrence of aspiration pneumonia has decreased in sedated ventilated patients who were being fed enterally.

Step 2: Use the PICOT Method: Determine the Population of Interest

Patient or Population (P)

- Pediatric patients admitted to the PICU who are mechanically ventilated

Intervention (I)

- Placement of postpyloric feeding tubes for all mechanically ventilated patients

Comparison (C)

- Postpyloric feeding tubes versus gastric feeding tubes

Outcome (O)

- Decreased incidence of aspiration pneumonia in the PICU patients receiving long-term mechanical ventilation

Step 3: Identify the Team Members Involved

- Project leader: Maryann Godshall
- Six-nurse insertion team: Loretta Smith, Brenda Jones, Beth Sands, Jen Long, Pat Pine, and Maryann Godshall
- MD consultant: Dr. Kerrie Pinkney (intensivist)

Step 4: Develop a Timeline

9/20/07: First meeting
9/30/07–10/30/07: Gather evidence in literature
11/1/06–5/1/07: Study period
6/1/07: Project complete

Step 5: Identify Search Terms

- Postpyloric tube feedings
- Long-term tube feedings
- Gastric tube feedings
- Jejunal tube feedings
- Enteral tube feedings
- Aspiration pneumonia
- Transpyloric tube feedings

Step 6: Determine Search Engines

- CINAHL
- EBSCO
- OVID Online
- Cochrane Database
- PubMed

Step 7: Gather the Evidence and Prepare an Evidence Table

Table 11.1 presents the evidence compiled from just two of the research articles found for this project.

Step 8: Summarize Your Evidence

- The evidence shows that transpyloric feeding tubes can be placed by the blind method easily (<5 minutes) and successfully (88.7%) in the PICU.
- This method should *not* be used in the neonatal intensive care unit (NICU).

Step 9: Identify Practice Implications

- Transpyloric feeding tubes can be placed easily and successfully in the PICU.
- Evidence shows that transpyloric tube feedings decrease the incidence of aspiration pneumonia.
- To decrease the incidence of aspiration pneumonia in the PICU, transpyloric tube feedings should be implemented.

Author's note: This is just one example of an EBP project. You can tailor the process to meet your institution's needs. Not all institutions rate the evidence. If you do rate the evidence, there are numerous rating scales available for you to use.

EXAMPLE 2

Step 1: Come Up With the Idea

EBP Project: Implementation of a rapid response team in a community hospital

The interest in this topic evolved from working in the hospital and wanting to decrease the "code blue" events. Our team wondered if implementation of a rapid response team in our institution would decrease the incidence of respiratory and cardiac arrests in the adult population.

Step 2: Use the PICOT Method: Determine the Population of Interest

Patient or Population (P)

- Adult patients older than 18 years of age admitted to a community hospital

Intervention (I)

- Implementation of a procedure and education of staff in the process of calling a rapid response

Comparison (C)

- Incidence of "code blue" events before and after putting in place a rapid response team

Outcome (O)

- Decreased incidence and number of "code blue" events in the hospital

Table 11.1

Example of an Evidence Table

Reference	Purpose/ Hypothetical Research Question	Sample	Classification of Evidence	Method	Results
McGuire, W., & McEwan, P. (2007). Transpyloric versus gastric tube feeding for preterm infants. *Cochrane Database of Systematic Reviews, 2007*(3). doi:10.1002/14651858. CD003487.pub2.	Does feeding via the transpyloric route vs. the gastric route improve feeding tolerance and growth and development without increasing adverse consequences?	Eight studies undertaken from 1970s through early 1980s. Very low birth weight infants (less than 1,500 g). Only infants with growth appropriate for gestational age were used. Some of the infants on respiratory or ventilatory support were not included.	3A–systematic review of homogeneity of case-control studies	Randomized or quasi-randomized controlled trials comparing transpyloric vs. gastric tube feedings in preterm infants	No evidence of benefit of transpyloric feeding in preterm infants. There were adverse effects found, and therefore feeding preterm infants via the transpyloric route *cannot* be recommended.

| Joffe, A. R., Grant, M., Wong, B., & Gresiuk, C. (2000). Validation of blind transpyloric feeding tube placement techniques in pediatric intensive care. *Pediatric Critical Care Medicine, 1*(2), 151–155. doi:10.1097/001304 78-200010000-00011 | Blind insertion of transpyloric feeding tubes in pediatric intensive care is highly successful. | Children in pediatric intensive care without fundoplication, pharyngeal trauma, or gastric ulceration, whose intensivists requested transpyloric feedings. Patients who were hemodynamically unstable to tolerate the procedure and those who had an absent cough while not endotracheally intubated were also excluded. Patients were <17 years old. Average age was 0.73–198 months of age and weighed 3–70 kg. The diagnosis included post-op heart surgery ($n = 15$), respiratory failure ($n = 7$), septic shock ($n = 4$), coma ($n = 4$), traumatic brain injury ($n = 3$), airway maintenance ($n = 3$), and burns ($n = 2$). Sixty-nine percent were ventilated, 15.5% had pharmacologic paralysis, and 78.9% had continuous infusion of sedation. Tubes were nasally placed in 94.4% and orally placed in 5.6% of patients. | 2C–outcomes research | Prospective interventional study | Seventy-one feeding tubes inserted in 38 patients over a 9-month period from February 1999 to October 1999. Success rate of blind transpyloric feeding tube insertion was 88.7%. The average insertion time was 5 min. |

Step 3: Identify the Team Members Involved

- Project leader: Maryann Godshall
- Six-nurse team: Loretta Smith, Brenda Jones, Beth Sands, Jen Long, Pat Pine, and Maryann Godshall
  - ICU charge nurse: Becky Reid
  - Respiratory therapist: Kay Fritz
- MD consultant: Dr. Kerrie Pinkney, intensivist

Step 4: Develop a Timeline

1/20/15: First meeting
3/30/15–5/30/15: Gather evidence in literature
6/1/15–12/31/15: Study period
1/31/16: Project complete

Step 5: Identify Search Terms

Author's note: These teams are known by different acronyms at various institutions.

- Code blue
- Rapid response
- Rapid intervention
- Respiratory support
- Respiratory arrest (and outcomes)
- Cardiac arrest (and outcomes)
- Critical assessment team (CAT) calls

Step 6: Determine Search Engines
- CINAHL
- EBSCO
- OVID online
- Cochrane Database
- PubMed

Step 7: Gather the Evidence and Prepare an Evidence Table

Table 11.2 is a more detailed example of an evidence table.

Table 11.2

Example of a More Detailed Evidence Table

First Author/ Publication/ Year	Conceptual Framework	Design/Method	Sample/ Setting	Major Variables Studied (and Their Definitions)	Measurement	Data Analysis	Findings	Appraisal: Worth to Practice
Chan, P. S., et al. (2010). *Archives of Internal Medicine, 170* (1), 18–26	None	SR Purpose: effect of RRT on HMR and CR ■ Searched five databases from 1950 to 2008 and "gray literature" from MD conferences ■ Included only 1. RCTs and prospective studies with 2. A control group or control period and	$N = 18$ of 143 potential studies Setting: acute care hospitals; 13 adult, 5 peds Average no. beds: NR Attrition: NR	IV: RRT DV1: HMR (including DNR, excluding DNR, not treated in ICU, no HMR definition) DV2: CR	RRT: Was the MD involved? HMR: overall hospital deaths (see definition) CR: cardiac and/or pulmonary arrest; cardiac arrest calls	■ Frequency ■ Relative risk	13/16 studies reporting leam structure 7/11 adult and 4/5 peds studies had significant reduction in CR CR: ■ In adults, 21%– 48% reduction in CR: RR 0.66 (95% CI, 0.54–0.80)	Weaknesses: ■ Potential missed evidence with exclusion of all studies except those with control groups ■ Gray literature search limited to medical meetings ■ Only included HMR and CR outcomes ■ No cost data

(continued)

Table 11.2

Example of a More Detailed Evidence Table (continued)

First Author/ Publication/ Year	Conceptual Framework	Design/Method	Sample/ Setting	Major Variables Studied (and Their Definitions)	Measurement	Data Analysis	Findings	Appraisal: Worth to Practice
		3. Hospital mortality well described as outcome ■ Excluded five studies that met criteria due to no response to email by primary authors					■ In peds, 38% reduction in CR: RR 0.62 (95% CI, 0.46–0.84) HMR: ■ In adults, HMR RR 0.96 (95% CI, 0.84–1.09) ■ In peds, HMR RR 0.79 (95% CII, 0.63–0.98)	Strengths: ■ Identified number of activations of RRT/1,000 admissions ■ Identified variance in outcome definition and measurement (e.g., 10 of 15 studies included deaths from DNRs in their mortality measurement) Conclusion: ■ RRT reduces CR in adults and CR and HMR in peds

Citation		Design/Purpose	Sample	Variables	Measures	Statistic	Findings	Appraisal
McGoughey, J., et al. (2007). *Cochrane Database of Systematic Reviews, 3*, CD005529	None	SR (Cochrane review) Purpose: effect of RRT on HMR ■ Searched six databases from 1990 to 2006 ■ Excluded all but two RCTs	*N* = 2 studies. Acute care settings in Australia and the UK. Attrition: NR	IV: RRT DV1: HMR	HMR: Australia: overall hospital mortality without DNR UK: Simplified Acute Physiology Score (SAPS) II death probability estimate	OR	OR of Australian study, 0.98 (95% CI, 0.83–1.16) CR of UK study, 0.52 (95% CI, 0.32–0.85)	Feasibility: ■ RRT is reasonable to implement; evaluating cost will help in making decisions about using RRT ■ Risk–benefit (harm): benefits outweigh risks Weaknesses: ■ Did not include full body of evidence ■ Conflicting results of retained studies, but no discussion of the impact of lower level evidence Recommendation: ■ Needs more research Conclusion: ■ Inconclusive
Winters, B. D., et al. (2007). *Critical Care Medicine, 35*(5), 1238–1243	None	SR Purpose: effect of RRT on HMR and CR ■ Searched three databases from 1990 to 2005	*N* = 8 studies. Average number of beds: 500	IV: RRT DV1: HMR DV2: CR	HMR: overall death rate CR: number of in-hospital arrests	Risk ratio	HMR: ■ Observational studies, risk ratio for RRT on HMR, 0.87 (9.5% CI, 0.73–1.04)	Strengths: Provides comparison across studies for ■ Study lengths (range, 4–82 months) ■ Sample size (range, 2,183–199,024)

(continued)

Table 11.2.

Example of a More Detailed Evidence Table (*continued*)

First Author/ Publication/ Year	Conceptual Framework	Design/Method	Sample/ Setting	Major Variables Studied (and Their Definitions)	Measurement	Data Analysis	Findings	Appraisal: Worth to Practice
		■ Included only studies with a control group	Attrition: NR			Risk ratio	■ Cluster RCTs, risk ratio for RRT on HMR, 0.76 (95% CI, 0.39–1.48) CR: ■ Observational studies, risk ratio for RRT on CR, 0.70 (95% CI, 0.56–0.92) ■ Cluster RCTs, risk ratio for RRT on CR, 0.94 (95% CI, 0.79–1.13)	■ Criteria for RRT initiation (common: respiratory rate, heart rate, blood pressure, mental status change; not all studies, but noteworthy: oxygen saturation, "worry") ■ Includes ideas about future evidence generation (conducting research)—finding out what we do not know Conclusion: ■ Some support for RRT, but not reliable enough to recommend as standard of care

CI, confidence interval; CR, cardiopulmonary arrest or code rates; DNR, do not resuscitate; DV, dependent variable; HMR, hospital-wide mortality rates; IV, independent variable; NR, not reported; OR, odds ratio; peds, pediatric patients; RCT, randomized controlled trial; RR, relative risk; RRT, rapid response team; SR, systematic review; UK, United Kingdom.

Source: Adapted from Fineout-Overholt, C., Melnyk, B. M., Stillwell, S. B., & Williamson, K. M. (2010). Evidence-based practice, step by step: Critical appraisal of the evidence: Part III. *American Journal of Nursing, 110*(11), 43–51. doi:10.1097/01.NAJ.0000390523.99066.b5

Step 8: Summarize Your Evidence

- The evidence shows that implementing a rapid response team decreased cardiac arrests in one study, but it was inconclusive in the other study. More research is needed.

Step 9: Identify Practice Implications

- Additional evidence should be evaluated to see if implementing a rapid response team has more favorable outcomes.
- A rapid response team should be implemented and research conducted in our institution to monitor whether the incidence of "code blue" is decreased.
- Findings should be discussed with the "code blue" team, followed by brainstorming after reviewing the evidence, to identify different ways that may be more effective for utilizing rapid response teams to prevent the progression of patients to a full "code blue" status in our institution.

Glossary

Abstract A brief summary about the research article. It should contain the purpose, methods, and major findings of the study. By reading an abstract, the researcher should be able to understand the basic highlights of a research article.

Aesthetic knowledge Abstract information that gives us an appreciation of the deeper meaning of the situation. It takes an inductive approach to knowledge acquisition.

Assumptions Statements and principles that are taken as truth, based on a person's values and beliefs.

Bias Occurs when researchers interject their personal beliefs into the study. This is a deviation from the true results of the study.

Biophysiological measure A measure that includes both in vivo and in vitro measures. A biophysiological method is one that tests an instrument of some kind.

Bivariate study A study with two variables. One variable is usually the dependent variable, and the other is the independent variable.

Blinding Occurs during the research process when the subjects do not know if they are in the experimental group or the control group.

Boolean operators Words that are used to connect or exclude key words in a search. These produce a more focused result.

Borrowed theories Theories taken from another discipline, for example, psychology, and applied to nursing questions and research problems.

Bracketing The process by which researchers identify their own personal biases about the phenomenon of interest to clarify their personal experiences and beliefs that may alter or reflect what is heard and reported.

Case studies In-depth examinations of people or groups of people. In a case study, institutions or facilities could be examined, for example, an inpatient psychiatric unit.

CINAHL (Cummulative Index of Nursing and Allied Health Literature) Largest and most in-depth nursing database. First published in 1961, it covers nursing and allied health journals, including dental hygiene, nutrition, occupational therapy, physical therapy, physician assistant, and respiratory therapy journals. It is an index to print and online articles.

ClinicalKey A database that provides full-text access to journals, textbooks, articles, practice guidelines, patient handouts, and drug information.

Clinical practice guidelines Systematic reviews that put a large amount of evidence into a manageable and usable format. They give specific practice recommendations for making evidence-based practice (EBP) decisions, address the issues relevant to a clinical decision, which include balancing the benefit and risks of an EBP decision, and are developed to help guide clinical practice even when there is limited available evidence.

Cochrane Database of Systematic Reviews One of the most popular databases in the Cochrane library that provides systematic reviews of current research.

Community-based participatory action research A method of research that involves the community to take an active part in all stages of the research process, including planning, conducting, implementing, and evaluating.

Comparative studies Studies that look at the difference between intact groups on some dependent variable of interest.

Comparison Occurs when an individual assesses the similar and dissimilar characteristics of a particular object, situation, or research variable.

Concepts The building blocks of theories that are used to describe a phenomenon or a group of phenomena. A concept gives some degree of classification or categorization.

Conceptual model In research, similar to a conceptual framework. It is a set of abstract and general concepts that are assembled to address a phenomenon of central interest.

Confidence intervals Reflect the degree of risk researchers are willing to take of being wrong. With a 95% confidence interval, researchers accept the probability that they will be wrong only 5 times out of 100.

Constructs Higher level concepts that are derived from theories and that represent nonobservable behaviors.

Control or comparison group The group not receiving the intervention of interest, or the group with which the experimental group is compared.

Correlational studies Studies in which the researcher examines the strength of the relationship between variables by determining how the change in one variable is associated with the changes in another variable.

Cross-sectional A survey or study that looks at people at one point in time.

Database A collection of data or information stored in a computer. You can think of it as an electronic filing system.

Dependent variable The "effect" or that which is influenced by the independent variable. The dependent variable can also be called the criterion, or outcome variable.

Descriptive studies Studies that describe things or objects, the phenomena of interest, or the relationship between variables. This is different from an exploratory study in that there would be information in the literature about the phenomena of interest in a descriptive study.

Descriptive theory Empirically driven theory that describes or classifies specific characteristics or aspects of individuals, groups, situations, or events by summarizing items in common that are found by direct observations.

Directional hypothesis Shows that there is an expected direction in the relationship between variables.

Double blinding A two-way process in which neither the researcher nor the subject knows who received the intervention and who is in the control group in a study.

Effect size The magnitude of the impact of an intervention or variable is expected to have on the outcome.

Emic Intrinsic or from the internal perspective of a culture.

Empirical data Documented evidence or data obtained through direct observation versus a subjective belief.

Empirical knowledge What we know through our physical senses; something we can hear, touch, taste, and see. Investigations of these areas are best handled through quantitative methods of knowledge discovery.

Ethical knowledge That by which we make moment-to-moment decisions: what is right, what should be done, and what is good. This type of knowledge directs our personal conduct in life.

Ethnography A qualitative study that explores the cultural aspects of a particular group of informants.

Ethnonursing A qualitative study that explores the cultural aspects of a particular group of informants in relation to nursing or how they perceive aspects of nursing care.

Etic Extrinsic, or from the external perspective of a culture.

Evidence-based medicine (EBM) The use of research-based information to make decisions about patient care delivery and practice of medicine.

Evidence-based practice (EBP) The use of research-based information in making decisions about patient care practice, paying attention to individual and group needs.

Experimental group The group of subjects receiving the intervention of interest.

Explanatory research studies Studies in which the researcher searches for causal explanations. This method is much more rigorous than exploratory or descriptive research. The researcher provides an explanation for the relationships that are found between the phenomena.

Explode A technique used to expand a database search to include other terms. This is done by including additional narrower subject headings in the key word list.

Exploratory studies Studies conducted when little is known about the phenomena.

Extraneous variables Variables that are not under investigation or examination but may (or may not) be relevant to or interfere with the study. Extraneous variables may be controlled or uncontrolled by the researcher. The researcher should identify any extraneous variables when possible to avoid interference with the study or the occurrence with any adverse or unplanned effects. Extraneous variables may also be called *confounding variables*, *intervening variables*, or *mediating variables*.

Feminist research Research that focuses on gender domination and discrimination within patriarchal societies. These researchers seek to establish a nonexploitive relationship with their informants and to conduct research that transforms these perceived boundaries.

Field notes Notes the researcher may take about an interview to help to remember facts that were important to the study (usually done after the interview is completed).

Focus Technique used to narrow a search when using certain computer databases.

Grand theories Complex and broad in scope. They try to explain broad areas and include many concepts that are not usually grounded in empirical data (data gathered through the senses using objective measurement) or evidence.

Grounded theory A qualitative approach in which a theory is developed that is grounded in the data obtained from research studies in which data is collected and analyzed.

Hawthorne effect Occurs when the subjects in a study change their behavior, actions, or answers to questions because they know they are being studied. They may answer a question the way they think the researcher wants it answered as opposed to how they really feel.

Health Insurance Portability and Accountability Act (HIPAA) of 1996 A law passed by the U.S. Congress that created national standards for maintaining the privacy of electronic medical information. An institution, such as a hospital, can disclose individually identifiable health information (IIHI) from its records if a patient signs an authorization gaining access.

Hyperlink A link (in the form of a web address or words in a text document) that automatically connects a computer (links it) with an item of interest that is accessible online. Hyperlinks are used to make access to online information easier.

Hypothesis In research, a prediction about the relationship between two or more variables.

Immersion A research technique in which the researcher spends time at the place of interest so that the participants or informants gain trust in the researcher or simply get to know the researcher, enabling more open discussions.

Independent variable The "cause," or the variable that influences the dependent variable.

Index Medicus The best known index of medical literature, first published in 1879. Although still available on library shelves, print publication ceased in December 2004 with volume 45. In 1997 this database became available for free on the Internet through MEDLINE.

Instrument A device or piece of equipment that measures a concept or variable of interest.

Instrumental case study Used when a researcher is pursuing insight into an issue or wants to challenge some generalization and the particular case was instrumental or of utmost importance to the subject being studied.

Integrative review A scholarly paper that synthesizes published studies and articles to answer questions about a phenomenon of interest; this type of review is frequently found in peer-reviewed professional publications. It provides generalizations about substantive issues from a set of studies that have direct bearing on those issues.

Interrater reliability The degree to which two or more individuals, or "coders," gathering information during a study agree. For judging purposes, it is a consensus, or how often they agree on a given score. In research, it is how often two observers agree on a given item and the level of agreement between them.

Intervention An action that is performed with the defined patient population. A nursing intervention is a nursing measure that is physically done to a patient.

In vitro A measure taken from a participant in a study and then subjected to laboratory analysis, such as the measuring of a potassium level, bacterial count, or a tissue biopsy.

In vivo A measure that is performed directly within or on a living being. (Examples include blood pressure, heart rate, and respiratory rate.)

Key informant A person who is knowledgeable about the population of interest to a researcher. He or she might also be able to provide the researcher with access to the designated population.

Key words Terms that describe the subject of interest in a research study.

Knowledge-focused trigger Idea that comes from staff when they listen or read research presentation or encounter EBP guidelines. It triggers an idea based on knowledge.

Landmark studies Studies that may have been published more than 5 years ago but are considered paramount to the direction of study of a particular topic. These studies are significant to the understanding of the topic.

Letter of query A letter sent to the members of the editorial board of a journal or magazine, asking if they would be interested in evaluating an article for possible publication.

Level of significance A measure of how much evidence a researcher has collected against the null hypothesis. It is written as a probability value, or p value. If the p value is less than 0.05, the result is significant. If the p value is greater than 0.05, the result is not considered significant.

Limitations Parts of a study that may confound or interfere with the main study variables.

Literature review A summary of the most important and scholarly literature on a particular topic.

Lived experience The focus of phenomenology that consists of everyday experience of a person in normal daily living.

Longitudinal survey or study A study that follows subjects over a period of time.

MEDLINE The largest searchable database that covers medicine, health, and research.

Meta-analysis The process of combining results of studies into a measurable format, statistically estimating the effects of proposed interventions, and critically reviewing them to minimize bias.

Metaparadigm A primary phenomenon of interest to a particular discipline. The nursing metaparadigm usually consists of four components: the person, the environment, health, and how the concept of nursing fits into the metaparadigm.

Methodological studies Studies in which the researchers look at the method; these studies are used mainly to test instruments or look at the development, testing, and evaluation of research instruments.

Middle range theories Theories that focus on only a piece of reality or human experience, involving a selected number of concepts, such as theories of stress.

Narrative research A type of research that allows people to "tell their own stories" to uncover their motivations, desires, or feelings in a multitude of settings.

Nondirectional hypothesis Shows no direction between the variables studied.

Null hypothesis Complete lack of or absence of a relationship between the variables studied.

Nursing Studies Index (NSI) An annotated guide to English-language reports of studies and historical and bibliographical materials about nursing. It is helpful when looking for material published during the first half of the 20th century (1900–1959).

Outcome The end result. What one wants to accomplish or measure.

Peer-reviewed journal A journal in which all articles are reviewed by experts in the field of the research topic. An article must pass the test of usually more than one expert or reviewer before it is accepted for publication. The review process usually takes place in a blinded fashion, in which reviewers do not know the author. All identifying author criteria and credentials are omitted from the article prior to the review process.

Personal knowledge The shared human experience and humanistic qualities of knowing. It concerns our inner experience.

Phenomenology A method that explores the meaning of human experience through the "lived experience" of the individual.

PICOT Five components that provide a structure when coming up with a clinical question (P—Patient, I—Intervention, C—Comparison, O—Outcome of interest, and T—Time frame to complete the project).

Pilot study A small-scale trial run of a larger research study, usually using a smaller number of subjects.

Population The group of individuals a researcher wants to examine. It can be infants, toddlers, preschoolers, adolescents, or adults of a particular age. It can also be a group of individuals, such as psychiatric patients with the diagnosis of schizophrenia.

Practice theories More specific than middle range theories, these theories produce specific directions or guidelines for practice. An example is the theories of end-of-life decision making.

Prescriptive theories Theories that address nursing therapeutics and the outcomes of interventions. A prescriptive theory includes propositions that call for change and predict the consequences of a certain strategy for nursing intervention.

Primary data sources Eyewitness accounts from the time being studied. Research studies by people who were actually present or the person who conducted the research or wrote about it.

Problem-focused triggers Ideas that emerge from issues noticed by staff in a clinical context to drive quality improvement or as a result of recurring clinical situations.

Problem statement A sentence that formally addresses the problem being examined. It is the "what" of the study. It should include the scope of the research problem, the specific population being studied, the independent and dependent variables, and the goal or question the study is trying to answer. It can be in the form of a declarative statement or an interrogatory question.

Purpose statement The reason the problem is being examined. It is the "why" of the study.

Purposive sampling A sampling method in which researchers use their own judgment in selecting people who will be representative of the group that the researcher is interested in exploring. For example, the researcher may go to a battered woman's shelter to study the lived experience of abusive relationships.

Qualitative research Research that is considered *subjective* and is more flexible in design. It describes an individual experience. It usually has a written narrative or verbal description. There usually are fewer participants in the study sample.

Quantitative research A type of research that is *objective*, imposes tight control over the research situation, and often has a rigorous and controlled design. It generalizes findings and frequently includes numbers, facts, and figures. When you think of quantitative research, think quantity. The sample study usually has a large number of participants or subjects.

Quasi-experimental design Similar to an experimental design except that there is no randomization or comparison group.

Query letter A letter of interest written to an editor to submit an article for publication.

Questionnaire A structured survey or set of questions that is self-administered or where an interviewer asks questions about a subject.

Randomization A procedure that assures that every subject has an equal chance of being chosen for the experiment.

Randomized control trial (RCT) The strongest type of evidence that is an prospective study evaluating the effectiveness of an intervention or treatment of a large sample of subjects.

Referred journal A journal that determines whether manuscripts will be accepted and published based on the recommendations of peer reviewers.

Reliability The ability to measure what one wants to measure on subsequent experiences.

Replication The ability for the researcher to repeat a study using the same design, method, and variables with very slight variations.

Research critique A critical appraisal or evaluation of a research project.

Research problem An area of concern or in which there may be a gap in knowledge or literature that is in need of a solution.

Research questions Statements of the specific query or investigation to answer or address a research problem. In some cases, they are a direct rewording of the statement of purpose, which is then phrased as a question.

Research utilization Application of a single research study or part of a study to something unrelated to the original research.

Retrospective study A study that looks backward in time to data already obtained and on record. This type of study can be done by reviewing charts of previously collected data.

Saturation A point that is reached when common themes are found in qualitative research and no new information is obtained. This is called the point of saturation.

Search engine An information retrieval system that is stored on a computer system such as the World Wide Web. One of the most popular today is Google.

Secondary data sources A view or account of an event by someone other than an eyewitness.

Scope In a searchable database, represented by an icon [■] that enables you to check the scope of a term and its synonyms.

Single blinding A one-way process in which subjects do not know if they are in the experimental group or the control group.

Standard deviation Shows the average amount of deviation of values away from the mean. A standard deviation is a useful variability index for describing a distribution and interpreting individual scores in relation to other scores in the sample.

Survey A method of collecting data to describe, compare, or explain knowledge, beliefs, or behaviors.

Systematic review A state-of-the-art summary of all the research information available at a given time on a particular subject. This is not a literature review but a review of actual research studies. Items in a systematic review all address a specific clinical question.

Truncation Used to find words with a similar stem and variant word endings. A common symbol of truncations is the asterisk (*).

Univariate study A study with just one variable.

Validity The ability of an instrument to measure what it is supposed to or intended to measure.

Variable A measureable characteristic that varies among the subjects being studied.

Vulnerable subjects Special groups of people in a research study whose rights need to be protected because they are unable or incapable of providing an informed consent. Examples include children, unconscious adults, mentally retarded or emotionally disabled people, severely ill or physically disabled people, or people who are terminally ill. Pregnant women are included because of possible unintended side effects to the unborn child, who is considered vulnerable.

Index

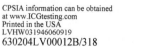

CPSIA information can be obtained
at www.ICGtesting.com
Printed in the USA
LVHW031946060919
630204LV00012B/318